GYNAECOLOGICAL
NURSING

GYNAECOLOGICAL NURSING

Maureen Reynolds

SRN, RCNT, DipN(Lond)
Clinical Teacher, Gynaecology
St Mary's Hospital
Manchester

Foreword by

Professor V.R. Tindall

MD, FRCOG
Department of Obstetrics
and Gynaecology
University of Manchester
Manchester

**BLACKWELL
SCIENTIFIC PUBLICATIONS**
OXFORD LONDON EDINBURGH
BOSTON PALO ALTO MELBOURNE

© 1984 by
Blackwell Scientific Publications
Editorial offices:
Osney Mead, Oxford, OX2 0EL
8 John Street, London, WC1N 2ES
23 Ainslie Place, Edinburgh, EH3 6AJ
52 Beacon Street, Boston
  Massachusetts 02108, USA
667 Lytton Avenue, Palo Alto
  California 94301, USA
107 Barry Street, Carlton
  Victoria 3053, Australia

First published 1984
Reprinted with corrections 1986

Set by DMB Typesetting, Oxford
Printed and bound in Great Britain
at The Alden Press, Oxford

DISTRIBUTORS

USA
  Blackwell Mosby Book Distributors
  11830 Westline Industrial Drive
  St Louis, Missouri 63141

Canada
  The C.V. Mosby Company
  5240 Finch Avenue East
  Scarborough, Ontario

Australia
  Blackwell Scientific Publications
    (Australia) Pty Ltd
  107 Barry Street
  Carlton, Victoria 3053

British Library
Cataloguing in Publication Data

Reynolds, Maureen
  Gynaecological nursing.
  1. Generative organs, Female—
  Diseases   2. Gynecologic nursing
  I. Title
  618.1′0024613   RG101

  ISBN 0-632-00963-2

Contents

Foreword

When asked to express an opinion about a textbook on gynaecology for nurses, I said it should be written by a nurse with considerable practical experience who was also a good teacher. This was because of my belief that nurses are essential for the smooth running of general and special gynaecological clinics, gynaecological wards and day case or minor gynaecological surgical units.

All nurses, even those in training, are expected by patients to know everything about gynaecological, sexual and marital problems or anxieties. Nurses are also expected to have knowledge of common obstetrical and post partum problems. It is essential, therefore, that the textbook covers all these aspects in a clear and sympathetic manner with examples of the type of problem which may be encountered.

It is a great pleasure to record that Maureen Reynolds has succeeded in this difficult task of providing the necessary factual and practical knowledge based on clinical experience. She has also helped to provide the answers to so many of the very personal questions likely to be asked by gynaecological patients and their relatives.

V.R. Tindall

Preface

When asked by Blackwell Scientific Publications to review existing literature on gynaecological nursing it became apparent that there was a limited number of textbooks which place the emphasis on nursing care linked to gynaecological conditions. An attempt has been made with this book to present gynaecological conditions and the nursing care in logical sequence. It should be useful to all those interested in or wishing to specialise in this field, student and pupil nurses, nurses undertaking postbasic education, i.e., ENB course 225 in Gynaecological Nursing, and anyone concerned with women's health care and health education in today's society.

Maureen Reynolds

Acknowledgements

My thanks go to Professor V.R. Tindall of The University of Manchester, who generously gave his time to reading the manuscript and making valuable suggestions which improved the text; also for supplying some of the illustrative material. I am grateful to Dr E. Blanche Butler, Senior Lecturer in Cytopathology at SMH, for her advice on Colposcopic Examination and Dr G. Ward, formerly Research Registrar Urodynamic Unit SMH, for providing much of the information for this section. I would like to thank the staff of Blackwell Scientific Publications for all their help and Miss G. Campbell for seeing this work through from manuscript to bound book.

My thanks go also to Miss H. Miller, District Nursing Officer, Manchester Central Health Authority and Miss D.M. Turner, Director of Nurse Education, Manchester Royal Infirmary, to my friends and colleagues in the School of Nursing and St Mary's Hospital for all their help.

Finally many thanks to Mrs B. Forbes for typing and retyping the manuscript with such patience, Miss M. Sidaway for checking the final proof pages and of course to my family for their support.

Photographic work was carried out by the staff of the Medical Illustration Department, Manchester Royal Infirmary.

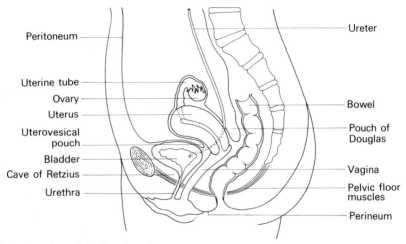

Peritoneum

Uterine tube
Ovary
Uterus
Uterovesical pouch
Bladder
Cave of Retzius
Urethra

Ureter

Bowel

Pouch of Douglas

Vagina

Pelvic floor muscles

Perineum

Sagittal section of the female pelvis.

1 The Role of the Nurse

Gynaecology is a highly specialized branch of medicine, it is not as is often thought simply another branch of surgery. Gynaecology is a subject which concerns itself with the most intimate and personal aspects of feminine existence. It concerns itself with issues that once were not even acknowledged let alone discussed, and which even now in an enlightened and ever progressive world are spoken of with hesitance, fear and ignorance by many. Deeply rooted ethnic and cultural beliefs persist in many communities which perhaps do not have ready access to modern services or knowledge. These factors and many others have a profound effect on gynaecology, and it therefore becomes clear that gynaecological nursing demands special skills of those who come to work in this field of medicine.

Women who seek advice or treatment on gynaecological matters may not always be able to present their case in a way which allows the problem to be defined, they may have a limited or distorted view of their own anatomy, they may, because they are embarrassed, choose words they feel they can use but which inaccurately described their condition. Of course not all patients fall into this category, many women are knowledgeable and articulate about their feelings and symptoms and present their cases well. Others are articulate but deliberately choose not to represent the real problem and as a result may confuse the clinical picture. Many patients fail to express their true feelings adequately, their true hopes or fears for the future.

If my definition of gynaecology seems sketchy this is because as well as being a study of the disorders and dysfunctions of the female reproductive system, gynaecology is also a science which inevitably includes endocrinology, urology, oncology and which by its very nature must include psychology and sociology to be complete. It is a fascinating specialty, for those who choose it there is great scope for developing skills acquired in training and acquiring new skills and experience as time goes on.

What then of the skills required to care effectively for the gynaecological patient? A patient may be seen in a variety of settings, i.e., clinic, ward or department. It is clear I hope from what I have said so far that a sympathetic approach is a prerequisite of good care and meaningful nurse/patient interaction. An ability to listen is of paramount importance and a mature outlook is essential on the nurse's part.

A patient who seeks advice, perhaps being referred to a gynaecologist by her general practitioner, will be seen at an outpatient clinic. Here she may present as hesitant, frightened, deceptively blasé or possibly even aggressive. It will take all of the nurse's skill in communication to adopt a reassuring attitude which will help the patient to overcome her fear of her environment or forthcoming procedures. It is at this point that the nurse can lay the foundation of a successful

1

examination, by getting the patient to relax and respond to preliminary question-ing. Sensitivity is obviously of great importance, patients are required to reveal many facts of an intimate nature, which, given the choice, they would prefer to keep to themselves. They are also required to reveal a major part of their anatomy which undoubtedly causes distress or at the least embarrassment. Brashness has no place in gynaecology, it would succeed only in making the patient feel uncomfortable, and effectively hindering or inhibiting communi-cation.

In this specialty powers of observation must be highly developed, the patient's demeanor, attitude and responses will reveal a great deal, and quite often a patient will confide in a nurse things she may not tell to a doctor because perhaps she is conscious of the demands on the doctor's time and the full waiting area outside the examination cubical. Or again it may be that what she has to say is so very personal.

The nurse in gynaecology has a unique contribution to make because she can appreciate so well the roles which her patient plays, i.e., wife, mother and especially the role of the female in today's society. This contribution will only assume full importance if the nurse has a good understanding of the structures and function of the female reproductive system and can relate this knowledge to nursing procedures.

Symptoms which the patient complains of will be of much greater significance if the nurse does take the trouble to understand gynaecological anatomy and physiology but also it will be easier to understand why psychological factors play so great a part in gynaecology. The patient who undergoes a hysterectomy, who suffers an abortion or is experiencing the menopause is not only experiencing physical disturbance but also mental disturbance. Depression is often experi-enced by gynaecological patients after surgery, especially in the early postoper-ative days. Guilt is frequently experienced by those who have a termination of pregnancy, and a feeling of loss of femininity may be suffered by women who have had ovarian surgery or a hysterectomy.

Infertility brings its own feelings of inadequacy and uncertainty about the future, marriages may suffer as a consequence of infertility and the sometimes interminable investigations which the couple undergo. There are of course many success stories which bring great joy.

In this chapter I have tried to give an indication of some of the emotional threads which run through this specialty. It is occasionally an emotive specialty but also may be quite common-place and straightforward. I have tried to suggest that the gynaecological patient may feel more vulnerable and 'emotionally' exposed, depending so much on a sympathetic approach and a very high degree of procedural and professional skill.

The nursing process is a means of achieving this high quality of patient care. It involves patient assessment, planning of nursing care, carrying out this planned care and evaluating the effects upon the patient. It is a means of giving individu-alized care to patients based on information obtained at the initial nursing assess-ment which is integrated and coordinated with the medical plan. I think it is

appropriate to list here some of the essential aims and objectives of gynaecological nursing care. I do not intend it as a definitive list, indeed it should be
added to as skills and experience become more highly developed.

AIMS AND OBJECTIVES

Aims

The aims of gynaecological nursing are to appreciate the physical, social and
psychological conditions encountered in gynaecological nursing, and be involved in the provision of appropriate nursing care and support needed by these
patients.

To give these general aims a sharper definition it is useful to provide a broad
framework of *general* objectives the achievement of which can be measured by
the use of *specific* objectives. As with all objectives, to be meaningful, they must
be expressed in behavioural terms.

Objectives

GENERAL

1 To assess the social, psychological and physical needs specifically required by
gynaecological patients.
2 To plan and manage immediate nursing care required by patients admitted to
a gynaecological ward for treatment whether emergency or elective.
3 To demonstrate an ability to carry out gynaecological nursing procedures and
evaluate the effectiveness of this care.
4 To discuss all aspects of gynaecological care including socioeconomic factors.

SPECIFIC

1 Relate knowledge of anatomy and physiology to gynaecological conditions.
2 Explain the psychological effects of diseases or disorders of the female reproductive tract.
3 Discuss the social, economic and psychological effects of gynaecological
conditions.
4 Communicate effectively with the patient and her family so that social,
economic and psychological needs are met.
5 Contact appropriate services, i.e., hospital, community or other agencies, to
secure help.
6 Recognize the profound psychological effects of certain gynaecological conditions suffered by some gynaecological patients.
7 Interview the patient to obtain data relevant to nursing assessment.
8 Prepare the patient for gynaecological examination.
9 Prepare the equipment and the environment.

10 Position the patient effectively for gynaecological examination.
11 Select appropriate instruments and speculae for gynaecological examination.
12 Assemble items required for cervical cytology.
13 Settle and comfort the patient following gynaecological examination.
14 Make adequate observation of the patient, and record.

INDIVIDUAL PATIENT CARE

Objectives which meet nursing care requirements of individual patients. The nurse will develop the ability to:
1 Prepare environment and equipment for the emergency patient.
2 Prepare for insertion and removal of a vaginal pack.
3 Perform vulval toilet.
4 Perform catheterization for retention or residual urine.
5 Perform wound dressings following major surgery, e.g., vulvectomy.
6 Remove perineal sutures.
7 Insert vaginal medications.
8 Insert vaginal dilators.
9 Manage and instruct the patient on bladder drill.

PREGNANCY DISORDER OR COMPLICATION

Objectives which meet the needs of patients admitted with a disorder or complication of pregnancy. Nurses must be familiar with the 1967 Abortion Act; it contains a clause that allows nurses to avoid all activity concerned with *procuring* of an abortion but which expects the nurse to give the necessary nursing care required by this patient. The nurse should be able to:
1 Describe the different classifications of abortion.
2 Demonstrate the principles of nursing patients who are threatening to abort.
3 Discuss the use of drugs which act upon the uterus.
4 Discuss the importance of diet in pregnancy.
5 Describe the use of drugs used in pregnancy.
6 Manage the nursing care of patient with hyperemsis gravidarum.
7 Discuss the various urine tests in pregnancy.
8 Prepare the patient for ultrasound and scan techniques.
9 Manage the nursing care of a patient following Shirodkar's suture.
10 Prepare the patient physically and emotionally for evacuation of the uterus.

INFERTILITY AND FAMILY PLANNING

Objectives which meet the needs of patients admitted for treatment for infertility or for family planning advice and treatment. The nurse should be able to:
1 Discuss the use of drugs in the treatment of infertility.
2 Discuss tubal patency tests and their significance.
3 Give adequate emotional support to patients undergoing tubal surgery for infertility.

4 Manage the collection of urine specimens for estimation of human chorionic gonadatrophic hormones.

5 Teach the patient to take and record body temperature relating to ovulation.

6 Explain the psychological effects of pregnancy.

7 Discuss the effects of conditions such as salpingitis and other infections in pregnancy.

8 Describe the main methods of contraception.

9 Advise the patient, and when appropriate, the partner or parents, on family planning.

10 Manage the nursing care of patients.

Lists of objectives, helpful though they are in defining gynaecological perspectives, are not intended to replace what essentially must be an individual and sympathetic approach to patients in the nurses' care. Each patient deserves to be treated as an individual for whom individualized care must be planned.

MODEL PREOPERATIVE AND POSTOPERATIVE CARE PLANS

To the care plan model, the nurse will add specific procedures which are appropriate to each individual patient. What is particularly important is that psychological needs as well as physical needs are met during hospitalization and convalescence. All patient care must be planned, and based on assessment, to achieve this end the nursing process provides a useful tool since the four components assessment, planning, implementation and evaluation allow individual and monitored care to be given to the patient.

It is wise to remember Florence Nightingale's remarks in her *Notes on Nursing* (1860) that a nurse must be primarily concerned with the person and not just the illness. Virginia Henderson's 14-point plan of basic individual needs concentrates on the *patient* rather than the medical condition.

The following care schemes relate in particular to the gynaecological patient, they must be used in conjunction with principles which are fundamental to surgical care. Many excellent textbooks are available which cover basic surgical care thoroughly, it needs no further mention here.

Preoperative

ADMISSION

Preferably admission will take place 24-48 hours prior to elective major surgery. The nurse will welcome the patient to the ward and check her identification. The patient's data should be confirmed, current medication checked, and the social and personal details noted. All medication and especially oral contraceptives must be noted on the Kardex and case notes as they are associated with venous thrombosis, and should have been discontinued 6 weeks prior to surgery. During this period of time the patient *must* be advised to use another form of contraception. Any possibility of pregnancy must be excluded, and, if necessary, a pregnancy test done. The nurse should then introduce the patient to the other patients and help her orientate herself to the ward. Finally, the nurse will outline the plan of care to the patient.

OBSERVATIONS

1 Base-line temperature, pulse, blood pressure and respirations.
2 Urinalysis.
3 Physical and psychological states.
4 Date of last menstrual period.

   These observations will accompany full medical examination by the doctor and in some cases the anaesthetist. At this point the patient's , and in some cases her husband's signature will be obtained by the doctor on the operation consent form. All operations which affect the woman's child-bearing potential, e.g., hysterectomy, oöphorectomy, sterilization surgery, will need the consent of the husband. Full explanations will be given prior to signing this form so that the patient and her husband fully understand what the proposed surgery entails, and what after effects there might be. It is the nurse's responsibility to check that the consent form has been signed and to reinforce the doctor's explanation. Further investigations will be arranged with relevance to the patient's condition and proposed surgery. They may include:

1 Full blood count; haemoglobin estimation; blood group and cross-matching, urea and electrolyte analysis.
2 Sickle cell test (vital in all non-Northern European women).
3 Mid-stream specimen of urine (MSSU).
4 High vaginal swab (HVS).
5 Chest X-ray.
6 Ultrasonography.
7 Electrocardiography (ECG).
8 Intravenous pylography (IVP).
9 Cystoscopy.

PREPARATORY MEASURES

Circulatory and respiratory systems

Preoperative physiotherapy and counselling will involve: breathing, pelvic-floor, mobility and leg exercises, and the discouragement of smoking with an explanation of why. These measures will encourage good preoperative and postoperative blood circulation and help to minimize the risk of chest infection.

Diet

The nurse must encourage adequate states of hydration (at least 2 litres in 24 hours) and nutrition in the patient. A low residue diet may be given in vaginal surgery. These measures will help to offset tissue trauma and fluid loss. The risk of an urinary tract infection will also be minimized.

Skin

The operation site has to be shaved usually the day prior to surgery. For abdominal surgery, the abdomen and pubis are shaved, and for vaginal and perineal surgery, the pubis, vulva and 'through' to the anus. The shave may extend to the midthighs if the patient is hirsute. Shaving for minor surgery is unnecessary but these procedures will help to minimize infection in major surgery.

When the patient has been admitted for elective surgery, she is able to bath herself, usually on the morning of the day of surgery.

Bowels

For bowel clearance: evacuant enema such as plain water, or phosphates in the form of a disposable enema. Bisacodyl suppositories are also useful. These evacuants should be given on the evening prior to surgery. These measures are necessary because of the proximity of the bowel to the uterus and vagina. Also defaecation can be avoided in the early days following vaginal surgery. Policies on bowel clearance vary from hospital to hospital, occasionally bowel preparation is omitted in minor surgery.

Vagina

Oestrogen creams or pessaries per vaginam may be needed preoperatively to improve vaginal tissue, especially in postmenopausal women. Packing of the vagina with gauze soaked in an antiseptic solution such as proflavine twice daily may be prescribed. These measures may be effective in treating local infection of the vaginal mucosa or cervical ulceration which may occur in procidentia.

Rest and sleep

Reinforcement of the doctor's explanations and correction of any misunderstandings will help to ensure rest. Night sedation will allow the patient to be physically rested. Rest is essential so that *stress* may be minimized. High stress levels are known to jeopardize postoperative recovery (Wilson-Barnett 1979).

Postoperative

POSITION OF THE PATIENT

On return to the ward, if the patient is fully conscious and there are no contraindications, i.e., epidural anaesthesia, she may be nursed in the dorsal position with one or two pillows. This has several advantages: pelvic drainage is encouraged, deep-breathing exercises are made easier, leg movements may be started, and fluids are taken more readily in this position.

OBSERVATIONS

Whilst positioning the patient, the nurse must carefully observe and record:
1 Wound drains.
2 Vaginal pack.
3 Indwelling catheter.
Other observations are directed towards recognition of haemorrhage and shock, these are initially half-hourly pulse, respirations, blood pressure and vaginal loss. If these vital signs are satisfactory and stable then 4-hourly recordings may be made together with continued estimation of vaginal loss and observation of any abdominal wound site.

PAIN

Each time observations are made the nurse must also make an assessment of the degree of pain. Analgesia is usually given immediately postoperatively by the anaesthetist. It must then be given as prescribed, whenever it is needed, which is usually 4-6-hourly for the first 24 hours following surgery. Analgesia is generally given via the intramuscular route and is often combined with an antiemetic if postoperative nausea or vomiting are troublesome. After the second day following surgery milder oral analgesia should be effective. Pain tolerance, however, varies from patient to patient.

URINARY OUTPUT

Many women find it difficult to void following pelvic surgery. The nurse should assist the patient to assume a position which she finds comfortable for voiding, a commode may be helpful, the sound of running water may also help. Usually micturition is possible within 12 hours.

It must be noted if frequent voiding of small amounts of urine occurs as this may indicate urinary retention with overflow. A distended bladder may pull on newly sutured pelvic tissues causing discomfort and possibly haematoma, therefore catheterization for retention must be carried out without delay. Some doctors prefer to commence continuous bladder drainage via an indwelling catheter for 48 hours until bladder tone is recovered, others advise single catheterization feeling that spontaneous voiding will occur afterwards. Another consequence of retention is a urinary tract infection. The patient must be encouraged to drink fluids so that stasis of urine is avoided; the aim should be 2-3 litres of fluid in 24 hours. A fluid intake and output chart should be maintained until the patient is drinking and voiding normally.

BLADDER DRAINAGE VIA INDWELLING CATHETER

The patient who has had vaginal surgery performed, particularly of the anterior wall usually returns to the ward with a Foley catheter *in situ* on continuous drainage. Occasionally if at surgery it was found that the bladder was firmly 'fixed', with adhesions, to the uterus and required extra handling and dissection to free it a Foley catheter may be inserted and continuous bladder drainage employed for 48 hours. This is to avoid retention which is likely if the bladder has been unavoidably traumatized at operation. Any indwelling catheter requires meticulous care and regular cleansing is essential, changing of drainage bags should be done using an aseptic technique.

When the catheter is removed (according to the surgeon's wishes) bladder drill may be instigated and the amount of residual urine estimated (see pp. 85 and 86). The patient will need extra support and reassurance at this point, often she will be so anxious to pass urine that quite the opposite is achieved.

VAGINAL PACKS

Vaginal packs are used particularly in vaginal surgery. Their purpose is twofold: to keep the sutured vaginal walls apart, preventing adhesions and to maintain haemostasis.

NB A vaginal pack may *obscure* haemorrhage for a time, and by pressure on the urethra cause retention of urine. Packs are usually removed after 24 hours, following removal a close watch must be kept on the amount of vaginal bleeding. The removal of the pack should be noted in the patient's records.

BOWELS

The nursing care aim is to prevent unnecessary straining by the patient during defaecation as this may damage newly sutured pelvic structures. Since the bowel is emptied preoperatively and the patient taking a light or low residue diet post-operatively defaecation is usually deferred until 3 days after surgery, when bisacodyl suppositories may be given so that constipation is avoided. If suppositories are ineffective a phosphate or olive oil enema may be given on the following day. Special care must be taken, when giving enemata, particularly if vaginal and perineal surgery has been performed. Any patient who is having difficulty with spontaneous bowel action is likely to be anxious and preoccupied, extra explanations and reassurance will help to relieve any fears which may be inhibiting defaecation.

Abdominal distension is extremely common following gynaecological surgery, it is due to partial stasis of the gut preventing gaseous escape per rectum. This build up of gas in the gut results in acute and distressing pain. Early mobilization of the patient and the administration of warm peppermint water is usually effective.

Vulval care is necessary for women who are likely to have some vaginal bleeding postoperatively. It is unusual for there to be vaginal bleeding following tubal or ovarian surgery but patients having vaginal and perineal surgery or hysterectomy may experience vaginal bleeding. Hygiene of the vulval area must be carefully maintained to discourage bacterial growth. Until the patient is fully ambulant and able to bath or shower, the nurse must perform vulval toilet for the patient at least twice daily.

The aim of vulval toilet is threefold: the maintenance of hygiene, the prevention of infection, and the soothing of any bruised or odematous tissues.

Procedure

1   Position the patient: dorsal with two pillows.
2   Expose only the vulval area.
3   Drape sterile towels over the patient's abducted thighs.
4   Using mild antiseptic lotion at 38°C swab the vulva thoroughly from front to back (towards the perineum).
5   With perineal sutures, turn the patient onto her side and swab the suture line.

Often the patient appreciates sitting on a bedpan whilst the antiseptic lotion is poured over the vulva and perineum. These areas must be thoroughly dried and whatever method used to cleanse the vulva a sterile pad is applied afterwards, secured in position with a belt or panties. This pad must be changed frequently.

SPECIFIC POSTOPERATIVE COMPLICATIONS

Haemorrhage

Haemorrhage is a serious complication of gynaecological surgery. If haemorrhage is excessive and goes undetected profound hypovolaemic shock will quickly result, the patient will have a rapid and feeble pulse, she will have a marked pallor and falling blood pressure which may be unrecordable. Anxiety is commonly seen in patients who are haemorrhaging and eventually because of a dramatic fall in circulating haemoglobin, *air hunger* is seen.

REACTIONARY HAEMORRHAGE

Reactionary haemorrhage occurs within the first 12-24 hours when the patient's blood pressure is rising as she recovers from surgery. A blood vessel which has been severed or a suture which slips from position causes bleeding. This bleeding may be seen if vulval pads are becoming saturated at each inspection or it may be intraperitoneal bleeding which is recognized by the patient's deteriorating condition. Excessive vaginal bleeding and other indications of shock must be reported immediately to the nurse in charge of the ward.

The safest treatment of reactionary haemorrhage is for the patient to return to theatre for religation of the bleeding blood vessel.

SECONDARY HAEMORRHAGE

A secondary haemorrhage is almost always due to infection and occurs 8-14 days after surgery. Amputation of the cervix and cone biopsy are both likely to cause secondary haemorrhage when sloughing has taken place and sutures have separated. Treatment is usually by packing of the vagina since sloughing makes resuturing difficult. The patient must be confined to bed until the bleeding has ceased.

The nurse must caution any gynaecological patient on discharge from hospital that she must report any bleeding per vaginam, and not assume that such bleeding is to be expected or that it may be menstruation.

Haemorrhage which occurs in vaginal surgery may be concealed in the form of a *haematoma* on the vaginal wall. This will be confirmed by vaginal examination and by the discharge of old blood several days after surgery. The patient will have complained of pain prior to this.

Deep vein thrombosis and pulmonary embolism

Deep vein thrombosis (DVT) is a 1-2 % risk in major gynaecological surgery. If a thrombosis does develop in the lower limbs there is a further risk of a massive and fatal pulmonary embolism if the clot becomes detached and is swept along to the pulmonary artery.

Factors which precipitate clot formation in the lower limb are:
1   The operative procedure.
2   Age.
3   Obesity.
4   Coagulation factors.
5   Vessel wall damage, i.e., varicose veins.
6   Preoperative and postoperative immobility.

It is now known that position is an important causative factor in DVT formation. The position of the patient in theatre, i.e., lithotomy, or continued pressure of the calves on the operating table and on the bed postoperatively. Calf stimulators used during prolonged surgery help to maintain a good circulation in the lower limbs.

Preventative measures begin preoperatively by encouraging mobility and then teaching the patient leg exercises as soon as she returns to the ward. Postoperative physiotherapy is vital and must concentrate on assisting the patient to be ambulatory within 24 hours when possible. Routine postoperative physiotherapy, which is a nursing responsibility is said to reduce the risk of fatal embolism fivefold. Sitting the patient by the bedside in itself is not sufficient exercise, in this position her legs are flexed and circulation is impeded. She must be helped to stand and take one or two steps. A TED antiembolism stocking may help to protect the patient from DVT, these stockings provide graduated compression to the lower limbs which improves venous flow.

Early recognition of a DVT is essential. The patient will complain of a pain in her calf and may develop a pyrexia. On examination her calf will be tender to touch.

Alimentary complications

Most women suffer from intestinal colic and slight abdominal distension after gynaecological surgery. They complain of 'wind' or gas pains which are most effectively dealt with by the nurse ensuring that the patient is:
1　Taking moderate amounts of fluids postoperatively.
2　Eating some solid food.
3　Mobilizing early.
4　Offered a peppermint mixture in hot water.

If abdominal distension is accompanied by severe and persistent vomiting, paralytic ileus is suspected and confirmed by an absence of bowel sounds. If this happens the patient looks anxious, her abdomen is tense and sore and she may be experiencing respiratory distress.

If vomiting is uncontrolled, dehydration, acidosis and electrolyte imbalance quickly occur. Myocardial infarction may be caused by potassium deficiency, although this is rare in gynaecological patients. Treatment consists of:
1　Analgesia and sedation.
2　Regular emptying of the stomach via a nasogastric tube.
3　Correction of fluid and electrolyte balance via intravenous infusion.
4　Maintenance of fluid intake and output chart.

Nothing is allowed by mouth until the return of bowel sounds indicates a return of peristalsis. Regular and frequent mouth care is necessary throughout this period.

Urinary tract complications

Most urinary tract complications are dealt with in the section on immediate postoperative care (pp. 8-9).

Urinary fistulae

When urine is found to be leaking from the vagina, this type of persistent incontinence indicates urinary fistulae caused by operative trauma or sloughing of repaired tissue. In ureteric fistula leakage will be into the abdomen. The proximity of the urinary tract to the reproductive tract makes fistulae formation between the two possible (see p. 75).

WOUND CARE

Abdominal wounds

Care of abdominal wounds follows the general principles of wound healing and wound management. Some wounds are left exposed others are dressed daily. What is important is that the wound is inspected regularly for signs of infection.

In gynaecological surgery pelvic contents are reached through a laparotomy incision or Pfannenstiel's (suprapubic) incision. In the latter technique the incision is transverse, usually along an elliptical skin crease. It heals well because being transverse less straining of tissue occurs and it also gives a good cosmetic result.

Many patients return to the ward with a fine polythene drainage tube in the subcutaneous tissue. This is attached to a collapsible plastic container (Redivac) which exerts a vacuum suction. By squeezing the sides of the container together air is expelled, this is then quickly attached to the drainage tubing, which should be clamped off during the procedure. Asepsis should be maintained throughout. The purpose of these drains is to prevent haematoma formation, they are usually removed after 48 hours when drainage has ceased. A nurse should be aware that the drainage tube is usually held in position by a suture which must be removed before removing the tubing.

Sutures and clips

Many types of wound closure exist from interrupted to subcuticular continuous suture to metal clips or staples. Tension sutures may be used for obese women or women with distended abdomens, i.e., carcinoma of the ovary. Removal depends upon wound healing but alternate sutures may be removed on the sixth day with the remainder on the seventh. Clips are usually removed on day 5 or earlier. If a wound is under stress, tension sutures may be left for 10 days or more.

Perineal wounds

Care of the perineum following surgery is mentioned on page 10. Catgut or Dexon absorbable sutures are used after perineorrhaphy but often they cause discomfort and need removal around the seventh day. Occasionally one or two of these sutures may dissolve and fall out which is alarming for the patient if she has not been warned of this likelihood and finds them on her pad.

ADVICE ON DISCHARGE FROM HOSPITAL

After major surgery

It is the nurse's responsibility to establish that the patient understands exactly the nature of her operation and how it will affect her body function in the future.

From the admission history, nursing staff should be aware of the patient's home circumstances and have assessed whether home facilities are suitable, or arranged supportive services to provide temporary additional help. If the patient is married, it is better, when possible, if the husband can arrange to take some time off work. This is not always feasible. Before discharge from hospital it is usual for the doctor to perform a vaginal examination, this will determine the presence of any haematoma and will also help to break down any adhesions which may have formed after vaginal surgery. If the woman is sexually active she will need advice on when she might resume coitus, this is usually within 4-6 weeks or after her postoperative check up in the outpatients clinic. Any prescribed medication must be continued as necessary and the importance explained to the patient. On the third postoperative day it is usual to check the haemoglobin and if it is necessary iron replacement will be commenced which may well be continued on discharge home.

Other advice must include avoidance of heavy lifting or strenuous exercises, light housework may usually be commenced after one month. Women usually appreciate specific advice on just what does constitute heavy lifting or light housework etc. The patient should continue with any regimens such as bladder drill or any established pattern of hygiene. She must also be reminded of the need to contact her doctor if she should suddenly start to bleed vaginally.

2 Gynaecological Examination

REASSURING THE PATIENT

Most women approach gynaecological examination with extreme reluctance indeed they may repeatedly postpone such examination and run the risk of allowing an abnormality to go undetected for a dangerously long time. The thought of having to discuss menstrual and sexual details may account for this reluctance or it may be the false impression that a gynaecological examination is painful. The nurse can do much to dispel these fears and embarrassments. An encouraging attitude will do a lot to put the patient at her ease and reinforce the feeling of having done the right thing in presenting for examination; as the possibility of future examinations is likely, one should not, by an insensitive attitude, jeopardize future examinations. Full explanations should be given to the patient on what a gynaecological examination entails.

Many patients fear that they may not be able to give precise details of their condition or they may fear misunderstanding all that the doctor says to them. The nurse can reassure the patient greatly by saying that she will be present during the examination and will listen to what is said in order to clarify anything which is not fully heard or understood at the time. This role of the nurse in gynaecological examination will both reassure the patient and prevent any information or instructions being misunderstood. The male doctor, who must be chaperoned throughout this procedure, will also appreciate this aspect of the nurse's presence during the examination.

The nurse can help to create an atmosphere conducive to good examination by ensuring privacy for each patient, and ensuring, by intelligent anticipation, that equipment likely to be used during the examination is readily available. The nurse cannot be merely a doctor's 'handmaiden' if she is to benefit the patient.

In examination it is for the nurse to call each patient without any undue delay to a prepared cubicle or examination room. The nurse offers the patient the opportunity to empty her bladder, as a prerequisite to gynaecological examination. A full bladder would obscure other pelvic structures, make examination difficult and make the procedure unpleasant and uncomfortable for the patient. Also, the nurse must explain exactly which articles of clothing to remove and how to wear an examination gown if so required. The nurse should anticipate the need for the patient to wear a protective pad if she is menstruating or has a vaginal discharge. (Information may be available about a patient since many are referred to a gynaecologist by their general practitioner/family doctor.) A patient should never be put in the embarrassing position of wandering around an out-patient clinic or department minus panties, tights or stockings. The sheer indignity of this might well ensure that the patient never returns.

If a particular patient seems unduly nervous or anxious it should be possible

15

without creating too much of an upheaval to see that she is seen by doctor at the earliest moment possible. Unnecessary delay should be avoided for all patients attending for gynaecological examination. This is difficult with busy clinics, but chaotic hurry should be avoided.

TAKING A GYNAECOLOGICAL HISTORY

A gynaecological examination cannot be done in isolation to the rest of the body. Obviously it must include examination of the other systems and organs of the body as, for instance, thyroid gland dysfunction or diabetes may effect a gynaecological disorder. It is for this reason that the nurse weighs the patient and performs a urinalysis directly before actual physical examination by the doctor, and that information pertaining to general health and body function is included in the history.

General medical details

Details of the following will be taken:
   Cardiovascular and respiratory systems
   Urinary system/bowel habits
   Family history
   Previous medical/surgical history
   Allergies or idiosyncrasies
   Weight gain or loss

Specific gynaecological details

Specific details should be obtained systematically and should include:
   Present symptoms or reason for examination, e.g., cervical cytology
   Age, occupation and domestic/social circumstances
   Menstrual details, i.e., menarche, menopause, menstrual cycle, last menstrual
      period (LMP) and the period previous to this
   Obstetric history
   Marital and coital details

The nurse should discreetly check that maximum privacy is ensured.

The examining doctor will avoid medical jargon when questioning the patient and usually starts with questions that allow the patient to answer promptly without undue hesitancy or embarrassment. Coital details will only be taken when the patient has relaxed. The patient must be allowed the time and opportunity to describe her symptoms and feelings in her own words.

Environment and equipment

The room should be comfortable and warm. The examination cubicle should have a couch covered by disposable paper sheets or drapes and a light blanket.

There should be good general lighting and an easily portable light which can be angled as necessary. There should be a footstool for the patient. Adequate receptacles are needed for soiled instruments and materials.

Pelvic examination often includes rectal examination and there should be equipment available to do this. The rest of the equipment should be conveniently placed within easy reach on a tray or trolley. It need not be sterile but must be either disposable or sterilized inbetween each use. Many hospitals or clinics have prepacked equipment supplied by the Central Sterile Supplies Department (CSSD). This greatly reduces the risk of cross-infection, especially from vaginal infections by trichomonal or monilial organisms.

PELVIC AND RECTAL TRAY

The following equipment should be prepared on the tray:

Gloves: assorted sizes and types
Lubricant/warm water
Sponge-holding forceps
Speculum (Sims', Cusco's, Fergusson's) of various sizes and disposable types
Wipes or swabs
Vulval pads

Equipment must also be available for cervical cytology, aspiration test, sponge biopsy and high vaginal swabs. This equipment is also assembled on a tray (Fig. 2.1):

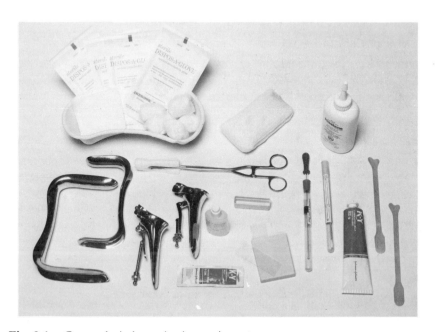

Fig. 2.1. Gynaecological examination equipment.

Glass slides and fixative slide carrier/container
Soft lead pencil
Ayre's spatulae
Pipette
Vulsellum forceps, sponge and sponge-holding forceps
Cytology request forms
High vaginal swabs (with appropriate pathology forms)

COLPOSCOPY

In many gynaecological clinics or departments a colposcope will be available. This instrument is used to examine the vaginal walls and the cervix under illumination and magnification. It enables the doctor to visualize these tissues when a previous smear has shown a suspicion of a cervical abnormality. With the colposcope the Schiller's test can be done under direct vision. In this test iodine is swabbed onto the cervix if there is an abnormal or malignant lesion the stain is not taken up because these lesions do not produce glycogen which is normally present and takes up the stain.

The great advantage of the colposcope is that the actual site of abnormality can be identified so that a biopsy may be taken for definite histology. Colposcopy rules out random biopsy and the risk of missing an area of abnormality. (See chap. 8.)

Positions

There are four different positions which a patient may be asked to assume by the doctor: dorsal, left lateral, Sims', and lithotomy. The nurse assists the patient as necessary.

Whichever position the patient is asked to assume adequate cover must be provided to prevent overexposure and subsequent tension which will make examination difficult for both doctor and patient.

DORSAL

For the dorsal position, the patient lies on her back with one pillow supporting her head. Her arms should be down by her side. After an abdominal examination the knees may be flexed and the thighs abducted (Fig. 2.2a). This position is used for bimanual examination as well as the initial vaginal examination and treatments requiring the insertion of Cusco's speculum. Vulval inspection is easier with this position.

LEFT LATERAL

The patient is asked to lie on her left side with her buttocks well towards the edge of the couch for the left lateral position. Her knees are flexed and her legs drawn up towards her trunk. Both arms are in front of her body (Fig. 2.3b). This

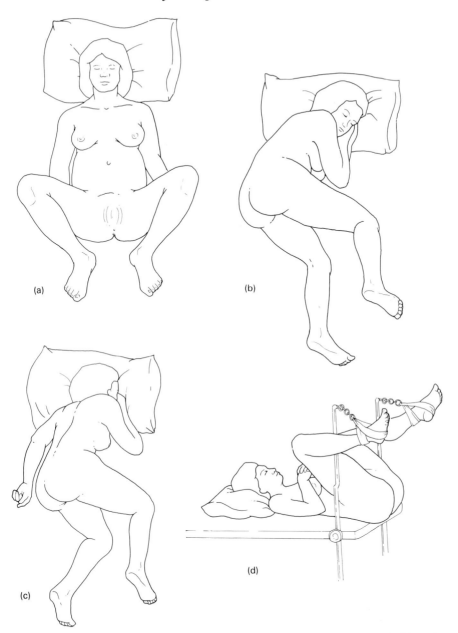

Fig. 2.2. Positions used in a gynaecological examination: modified dorsal (a), left lateral (b), Sims' (c), lithotomy (d).

is a comfortable position which encourages the patient to relax more. As the patient is facing away from the examining doctor, the nurse should, when circumstances permit, position herself facing the patient.

The left lateral position will facilitate rectal examination and may be used when a vaginal pack is inserted.

SIMS'

Sims' position is an exaggeration of the left lateral position. Here the patient lies almost on her front with her upper (right) leg flexed and her left leg extended. Her buttocks must be to the edge of the couch. Her left arm must be behind her but not uncomfortable (Fig. 2.2c). This position allows good visualization of the anterior vaginal wall, the abdominal contents fall forward in this position and when the Sims' speculum retracts the posterior vaginal wall the cervix can be easily seen.

This position is used for examining women thought to have a vaginal wall prolapse. The insertion of vaginal packs or pessaries is made easier by this position.

LITHOTOMY

In the lithotomy position the patient lies on a couch which is specially adapted to allow stirrups to be fixed to either side of the couch. The patient lies on her back, both legs are raised simultaneously and her ankles supported by straps which are fixed to the stirrups. Her buttocks are positioned to the end of the couch (Fig. 2.2d). This is a good position for performing cervical cytology but leaves the patient feeling very exposed so adequate covering should be available. This position is also used in vaginal and rectal surgery.

At the end of the examination the patient's legs must be lowered simultaneously, this, as with raising the legs simultaneously, is to prevent injury to the hips and back.

Physical examination

As I have said, the patient must empty her bladder before she is positioned. If a full colon is palpated, it is also misleading so occasionally examination has to be postponed until the colon is empty. As with history-taking, physical examination must be systematic or a vital clue to diagnosis will be missed.
1 *Firstly* the general appearance of the patient is noted: Is the patient anxious? Does the patient look ill? Are there any notable features, e.g., hirsutes, pallor?
2 The mucous membranes should be inspected for signs of anaemia.
3 The breasts should then be examined as they are part of the reproductive system and show changes, e.g., in pregnancy.

It is nurse's responsibility to see that the patient is appropriately covered during the various *stages* of examination.

ABDOMINAL EXAMINATION (DORSAL POSITION)

The nurse must know the sequence of the doctor's examination so that she can prepare and support the patient at each stage. She may recommend that the patient breathes in and out normally, as this may help her to relax.

1 Firstly the abdomen is inspected for obvious signs of striae gravidarum, scars or swellings, etc.

2 Then the abdomen is *palpated gently* to reveal any tender areas or masses. The pregnant uterus is felt in this way.

3 *Deeper palpation* will reveal abnormalities of the liver, kidneys and spleen, or the presence of a tumour, possibly ovarian.

4 *Percussion* of the abdomen may reveal tumours or ascites.

5 *Auscultation* with an ordinary stethoscope will determine the presence of bowel sounds.

PELVIC EXAMINATION

The patient remains in the dorsal position for the next part of the examination. Extra reassurance at this stage is timely. From the history-taking, the doctor will be aware of the signifance of virginity or nulliparity and will select a small speculum if the entrance to the vagina (introitus) is tight.

1 Firstly the vulva is inspected for redness, warts, lesions, discharge, soreness or swelling.

2 Perineal and anal regions will be inspected next. If the patient has had one child or more, old scars from an episiotomy may be seen.

3 The introitus is examined next. Enlarged Bartholin's glands or abscess may be noticed.

4 The vagina will be examined with a gloved index finger which is lubricated with some suitable preparation. Water is used if diagnostic tests are to be taken in order to avoid contamination.

5 Whilst the doctor's examining hand is palpating the vagina and cervix, he or she may place the free hand upon the abdomen and palpate pelvic structures at the same time to determine the outlines of the uterus, appendages, i.e., uterine tubes, ovaries or any pelvic masses. This is called a *bimanual* examination (Fig. 2.3).

6 Speculum examination is the next stage of the procedure. The patient may be asked to assume the Sims' (or left lateral) position if a Sims' speculum is to be used. The nurse will again assist and appropriately cover the patient, and may elevate the right buttock so that the vulva can be seen.

If a bivalve or Cusco's speculum is used, the patient usually remains in the dorsal position, but the Sims' (or left lateral) position can be used. The insertion of the speculum will be made more comfortable if it is slightly warm and lubricated. The Cusco's speculum is adjustable and self-retaining, which allows minor treatments and investigations to be carried out. Insertion will be made bearing in mind that the vagina runs upwards and backwards and that the urethra is in contact with the anterior vaginal wall.

One gynaecologist who has herself experienced speculum examination says 'If the speculum is inserted in the anterioposterior plane and then rotated the urethra feels as if it is being *scraped* by a steel blade'.

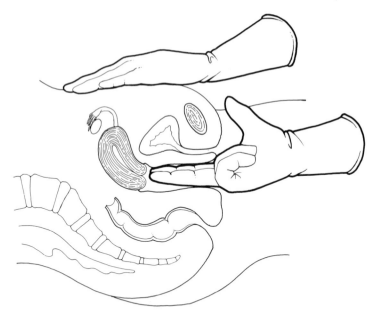

Fig. 2.3.   A bimanual examination.

During this examination the nurse can help the patient relax and if the doctor is intent on the examination and is not aware of the patient's questions, the nurse can respond and encourage the patient to defer her questions until the end of the procedure.

High vaginal swabs and cervical and vaginal cytology may be taken at this point. On completion of the examination the vulval and perineal areas must be wiped of excess lubricant or discharge. The patient is allowed to sit up and regain her composure. At this point the doctor and the patient may wish to discuss the outcome of her visit privately. One of the skills a nurse needs at a gynaecological clinic is to know when to withdraw to a discreet distance whilst such consultation takes place.

CERVICAL CYTOLOGY

If specimens are taken from the posterior vaginal pool or the cervix with the equipment outlined previously lubricants must not be used.

In 1943, Papanicolaou introduced a staining technique used to examine exfoliated cells to detect the presence of a malignant process. The material to be examined may be obtained by two methods:

1   Aspiration of the posterior fornix (pipette method). (Fig. 2.4a)

2   Cervical smear (Ayre's method). (Fig. 2.4b) A rotation of Ayre's spatula through 360° 'scrapes' exfoliated cells which can then be examined microscopically.

NB   'Pap' test is imprecise terminology relating only to a staining technique.

Before the specimens are obtained (usually by a doctor or a specially trained

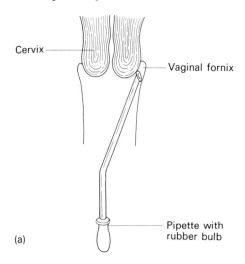

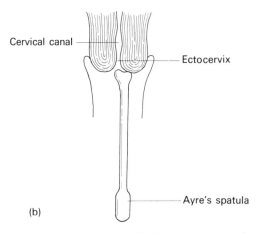

Fig. 2.4. Methods to obtain exfoliated cells from the cervix: the pipette aspiration method (a), cervical smear using an Ayre's spatula which is rotated through 360° (b).

nurse) the nurse should position the patient either in the dorsal or lithotomy position and reassure her that the procedure though it might be rather uncomfortable is painless. The nurse then prepares a glass slide by writing the patient's name and hospital/record number on the frosted portion of the slide, handling only the edges of the slide.

Once the specimen has been obtained, the nurse's role is as follows. The material obtained is transferred to the glass slide by gently smearing the spatula or contents of the pipette onto it. The specimen is then immediately fixed by placing a couple of drops of alcohol ether fixative onto the smeared specimen. The slide is then placed with the fixed specimen uppermost and allowed to dry before placing the slide in a slide carrier. Some centres simply place the glass slide directly into small containers of fixing solutions. Whatever method is employed the specimen must be carefully labelled as a mistake could prove disastrous.

Any specimens taken during examinations must be despatched to the laboratory with all the relevant clinical details on the accompanying card bearing the doctor's signature.

The nurse should make sure that before the patient leaves the clinic she is clear about her future appointment time and date. Most patients are likely to be anxious about the result of their cervical cytology tests. A patient can be reassured if she knows that the results will be available for her next visit to the clinic. The results may be sent back to the family doctor whom she may contact in 1-2 weeks.

NB   Any definite estimate of time should it be incorrect will create more anxiety for any women.

3 Common Gynaecological Problems

A gynaecological problem is often the reason why a woman first seeks medical advice. Often she is made to feel that what she is complaining of is trivial and that when she goes to her doctor she will be guilty of time-wasting. Any woman who suspects that she has a disorder or dysfunction of the genital tract should be positively encouraged to seek medical attention at the earliest possible time. The problem may seem trivial to her, but may well be a sign of a serious organic disease. Again, a reluctance to talk of these matters may be because of the embarrassment it might cause or because of a personal awkwardness in using the words to describe this condition.

Many a persistent vaginal discharge is ignored for months before the woman sees a doctor and it is discovered that the cause has been a malignant lesion of the cervix. Too often pruritus vulvae is tolerated for years, and a carcinoma vulva is diagnosed as the cause. As nurses we must take our share of the responsibility for improvement in health care of women, and recognize that many women need active encouragement to seek medical attention, regarding their problems.

Major gynaecological symptoms are discussed fully in their relevant sections. Here, the commoner problems which often prove quite simple to treat, are discussed. They are: dysmenorrhoea, premenstrual tension, dyspareunia, backache, and vaginal discharge.

DYSMENORRHOEA

Primary (spasmodic)

Dysmenorrhoea means painful menstruation. Young girls often complain of pain during menstruation, pain which they describe as intense and cramp-like. Several theories exist which may explain the origin of dysmenorrhoea which in this case is *primary* (*spasmodic dysmenorrhoea*).

THEORIES

Cervical obstruction

The theory of cervical obstruction was based on an idea that the cervical os was of pinhole size and impeded menstrual flow, a solution to this problem was to pass dilators into the cervical canal via this pinhole os. This procedure is rarely done these days as the outcome of this dilation was occasionally an incompetent cervix.

Uterine hypoplasia

Another theory that seems less valid today is uterine hypoplasia. It was thought

25

that an excessive amount of fibrous tissue impeded contraction of the uterine muscle.

Hormonal imbalance

Several hormone theories have been put forward to explain dysmenorrhoea but no conclusive evidence is available. It is however a fact that with anovular menstruation dysmenorrhoea is never experienced, which seems to support the theory that the balance between oestrogen and progesterone is responsible. More recent work suggests that the prostaglandins may cause uterine spasm.

Neurogenic factors

An imbalance or poor coordination of the autonomic nervous system is said to produce muscular spasm which may account for the pain. This theory fits well the image of a highly strung rather emotional girl. In primary dysmenorrhoea the patient is usually between the ages of 18 and 20. She may have menstruated for 2-3 years before this time but because it was anovular had not experienced pain. The pain occurs a few hours before and immediately after menstruation. It may be accompanied by nausea, vomiting or even syncope. The symptoms may be severe enough to result in regular time being taken off from school or occupation. Dysmenorrhoea of this type often disappears by the mid or late twenties and is invariably relieved by childbirth.

TREATMENT

Preventative

Preventative treatment is best based on curbing the intense spasm of uterine muscle and on avoiding repeated incapacitation. Girls must be adequately prepared for menstruation and the normality of this physiological function stressed. Preparation for menstruation should be comprehensively covered by each school's curiculum. The events which take place at the menstrual cycle should be explained fully. Practical advice should include the importance of regular bowel habits; constipation will aggravate dysmenorrhoea. Regular exercise will be beneficial. Social habits should be reviewed and fatigue and undue stress avoided.

Active

Active treatment should include advice on a good standard of general health, and diet. Whilst the pain is at its most intolerable the girl should be advised to lie down for a short while, some comfort may be derived from the application of heat to the lower abdomen. A mild analgesic may be helpful.

Drug therapy

The contraceptive 'pill' may be used with good effect, ovulation is suppressed and thus the pain. This treatment may be continued for 6 months after which the dysmenorrhoea may be much less when ovulation resumes. Progesterone only may be given to suppress uterine spasm this may be given in the form of dydro-gesterone (Duphaston) 10-20 mg from day 5 to day 25 of the cycle, or in the form of suppositories. Strong analgesia should at all times be avoided, drugs such as pethidine and morphine must not be used since regular use could lead to addiction.

SURGICAL INTERVENTION

Cervical dilatation

As mentioned under cervical obstruction, dilatation of the cervix with Hegar's dilators may be performed to relieve obstruction. If, however, the internal os becomes incompetent recurrent abortions may occur in future life.

Presacral neurectomy

The surgical procedure presacral neurectomy involves division of the presacral nerves. This is a major surgical procedure which is only undertaken when all other measures have failed.

Secondary, or congestive dysmenorrhoea

Dysmenorrhoea in women over 25 is generally associated with pelvic inflamma-tory disease or endometriosis. This is *secondary*, or *congestive dysmenorrhoea*. The pain is usually severe at the onset of menstruation and diminishes as the flow continues. Advice, as with primary dysmenorrhoea, is for women to take ade-quate rest at this time and mild analgesia. Any other treatment is based on treating the condition which is found to be causing the pain.

PREMENSTRUAL TENSION

The phenomenon of premenstrual tension (PMT) has recently attracted much publicity as within months of each other, two women were acquitted of criminal activities, with premenstrual tension cited as clinical evidence which mitigated the offences, offences as grave as manslaughter. This would seem to create a new legal precedent, which should stimulate further research into this condition.

Premenstrual tension is a collection of symptoms which are referred to as *premenstrual syndrome*. The symptoms are: irritability, insomnia, depression, dysmenorrhoea, lassitude, flatulence, abdominal bloating and migraine, or headache. Oedema is also a feature. The inability to concentrate is common as are extreme mood changes resulting in emotional outbursts. The woman appears to be accident prone and some of her abilities are impaired, e.g., driving. Research shows that the crime rate amongst women may be related to this distressing condition. Premenstrual tension also seems to be implicated in the suicide rates in women.

One patient thought to be suffering from PMT described her distressing symptoms in this way:

'During the middle of my menstrual cycle I become depressed and nervy, and approximately 10 days before the period starts the depression becomes acute. I get a sharp stabbing pain in the vagina and feel discomfort when sitting down. About 2 days before the period my depression is extremely severe. I often feel suicidal and am tearful. I am argumentative, easily lose my balance and in general do not know where to put myself.

I experience severe headaches and gain weight. My body is bloated.'

For married women, PMT can create a difficult situation within the family. Children will be bewildered by their mother's distress, and some husbands may be at a loss to know what to do. For single women sufferers, it is a time when understanding friends and relatives are much needed.

Causes

Salt retention is thought to be one of the major causes, which leads to fluid retention. This goes some way to explaining the oedema, the feeling of being bloated and mild cerebral oedema which might explain the menstrual migraine.

Excessive amounts of circulating oestrogen are also thought to be a causative factor, linked with the sodium retention.

Treatment

Any woman presenting with premenstrual tension will be fully examined to exclude a gynaecological abnormality or disease.

What this woman needs is a sympathetic hearing and it may be useful if her partner or a close relative is present for part of the interview to encourage more understanding of the condition. Many women have met rather curt and dismissive attitudes towards their syndrome, this merely exacerbates the issue. A logical explanation will go a long way to relieving the anxiety caused by the symptoms of PMT. A PMT chart (Fig. 3.1) is available for the patient to complete which can help in pinpointing when the symptoms increase and decrease in intensity. Advice to restrict salt and fluid intake may help to minimize the effects of PMT.

DRUG THERAPY

A *diuretic* such as frusemide (Lasix) 40 mg daily given 4-5 days premenstrual may minimize fluid retention.

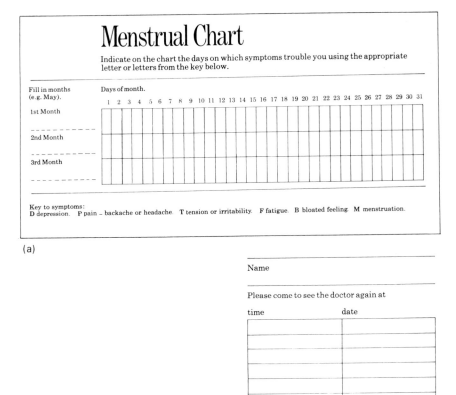

Menstrual Chart

Indicate on the chart the days on which symptoms trouble you using the appropriate letter or letters from the key below.

Fill in months (e.g. May).	Days of month.
1st Month	
2nd Month	
3rd Month	

Key to symptoms:
D depression. P pain – backache or headache. T tension or irritability. F fatigue. B bloated feeling. M menstruation.

(a)

Name

Please come to see the doctor again at

time	date

(b)

Fig. 3.1. A menstrual chart on which the patient can record the details of her premenstrual tension symptoms (a). The reverse of the card carries details of the patient's next appointment (b).

Progesterones may be tried to counterbalance the effect of excessive oestrogen, e.g., dydrogesterone (Duphaston). Hormones should be used only if other means fail. Progesterone suppositories cyclogest 200 may be used; one 200 mg suppository daily per rectum 2 weeks prior to menstruation.

Tranquillizers may be of benefit, and mild analgesia required for dysmenorrhoea and headache.

Antidepressants may be necessary in extremes of premenstrual tension.

DYSPAREUNIA

Dyspareunia is pain or difficulty experienced while involved in sexual intercourse. It may be superficial when the pain or difficulty is experienced at the vulva or introitus; or the dyspareunia may be deep and related to penetration. Dyspareunia may have pathological causes or may be psychological in origin.

Whatever the cause careful investigation is needed and treatment based on the underlying pathology. This is discussed in more detail in chapter 13.

BACKACHE

Backache, a more common gynaecological problem, may be caused by almost any gynaecological abnormality, but is frequently found to be of orthopaedic origin. Again treatment is of the underlying pathology.

Causes

UTERINE PROLAPSE

Laxity of uterosacral and cardinal ligaments may cause uterine prolapse or result in a retroverted uterus. Backache is a common feature of prolapse, or retroversion, because of displacement of pelvic structures.

CERVICITIS

Cervicitis of the chronic type probably affects the cardinal ligaments producing infection in these structures, and subsequent scarring from fibrosis which results in backache.

TUMOURS

Large tumours may, by their pressure on pelvic structures and their sheer weight, cause backache. Backache may also result from spinal metastases. As backache frequently emerges as a symptom of a gynaecological malignancy it becomes an important consideration in the planning of nursing care for a gynaecological patient, who is perhaps being nursed in the terminal stages of a malignant disease. Nursing care of a patient with backache should be planned with regard to maintaining good posture, either in a chair or in bed, which the patient finds comfortable. Extra pillows may provide good support and continual nursing assessment will enable positional changes to be made when needed. Analgesia should be given as prescribed by the doctor when required.

The old adage that 'if a woman says that she has backache then she has' is worth keeping in mind.

VAGINAL DISCHARGE

Vaginal discharge is probably the most common of all gynaecological complaints. A discharge may be normal or it may signify some underlying disease or condition.

Although the vagina does not have a secretion it is moistened by mucus from the cervical glands and a watery transudate through the vaginal walls. Therefore normal vaginal secretion consists of cervical mucus, watery transudate and desquamated vaginal epithelial cells. Also found in large numbers in vaginal discharge are Döderlein's bacillus (Lactobacillus). It is Döderlein's bacillus which is responsible for creating an acid media within the vagina. The squamous epithelial cells of the vagina produce glycogen and it is the action of the Döderlein's bacillus which converts this glycogen into lactic acid. A strongly acid reaction within the vagina produces protection against pathogens which may otherwise flourish in an alkaline media.

It is only in the menstrual years that the vaginal epithelium produces glycogen. Before the menarche and at the menopause there is a low output of oestrogen which affects glycogen production and therefore if there is little or no glycogen available for conversion by Döderlein's bacillus, the reaction of the vagina is alkaline. For a schematic representation of vaginal pH see Table 3.1.

Other commensals which live in the acidic media of the vagina but do not cause disease are *Streptococci, Staphylococci, Escherichia coli* and *Candida albicans.*

Diagnosis

The characteristic of a particular discharge may be suggestive of a diagnosis (Table 3.2) but definitive diagnosis is made by obtaining a drop of the discharge with a vaginal swab or platinum loop. This is then transferred to a glass slide and a little saline added. When examined under a high powered microscope pus cells can be clearly seen, squames are also seen and then a moving organism, *Trichomonas vaginalis* (Fig. 3.2a), can be easily identified. The trichomonads are a highly motile organism and the whip-like action of their flagellae can be observed.

If a specimen is similarly prepared from a patient thought to have a monilial infection, i.e., *Candida albicans*, the microscope appearance is different. Here fungus can be identified and in amongst the branching fungi, spores are seen (Fig. 3.2b).

The nurse's role in diagnosis of vaginal conditions will be to obtain a high vaginal swab and despatch it along with the pathology request form to the lab-

Table 3.1 Schematic representation of vaginal pH.

Vaginal factor	Premenarche	Maturity (menstruating years)	Menopause
Oestrogen	Low	Increased	Decreased
Glycogen	Low	Increased	Low
Döderlein's bacillus	Inactive	Active	Absent
pH	6-8	3.5-4.5	7-8
Reaction	Acid to alkaline	Acid	Neutral to alkaline

Table 3.2 Schematic representation of vaginal discharge.

Description	Causative organism	Condition	Treatment
White	—	Normal	Nil
White (increased)	—	Leucorrhoea—may be pathological, i.e., fibroids, endometriosis.	Good vulval hygiene. Treat the underlying cause.
White, scanty, curd-like and irritant	Candida usually *Candida albicans*	Thrush; candidiasis; candidal vaginitis. The discharge may be adhering to the vaginal walls, in rugal folds. It may produce extreme pruritis.	Investigate predisposing cause, e.g., diabetes. Nystatin cream or vaginal pessaries nightly for 2 weeks. Oral nystatin may be needed.
Green, profuse, frothy and very offensive also irritant	A protozoan *Trichomonas vaginalis*	Trichomonas vaginitis. Transmitted by sexual intercourse but can be spread via contaminated toilet articles. It is a sexually transmitted disease.	Avoid sexual intercourse. Metronidazole tablets 200 mg three times each day for 7 days. Alternatively Amphotercin B (Fungilin) vaginal pessaries may be prescribed. Also the sexual partner must be treated.
Purulent, occasionally offensive	Nonspecific, i.e., *Staphylococci*, *Streptococci*, *Escherichia coli*	Atrophic vaginitis or a foreign body, i.e., a tampon.	Gyno-Daktarin cream PV or dienoestrol cream (Ortho-Cilag) 1-2 applicators full daily for 1-2 weeks. Oral ethinyl-oestradiol 0.01 mg daily for one month. Remove foreign body.
Mucoidal, thick and slimy	Nonspecific	Chronic cervicitis Cervical erosion Cervical polypi	Treat cervicitus: diathermy or cryosurgery. Avulsion of polyp.
Bloodstained or brown	—	Carcinoma cervix Carcinoma uterus Cervical erosion Pregnancy (threatened abortion)	Treatment of underlying cause.

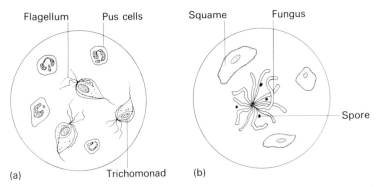

Fig. 3.2. Vaginal discharge infected with *Trichomonas vaginalis* (a) and *Candida albicans* (b).

oratory for culture and sensitivity. In counselling the patient, the nurse must include details for vulval hygiene. The patient should bathe or shower daily at least. Her underclothing must be fresh each day and if vulval pads are worn they must be changed frequently and if possible incinerated. The nurse must ensure that the patient fully understands how she is to use any prescribed medication. When patients are given inadequate instruction in the use of vaginal pessaries, it has been known for patients to take preparations intended for vaginal use, orally. **NB** Specimens, high vaginal swabs (HVS) are rendered useless if refrigerated. The most satisfactory HVS is obtained by inserting a Cusco's speculum into the vagina and obtaining material from the posterior fornix on a cotton wool tipped orange stick. This also applies to the method of obtaining material via pipette aspiration.

4 Gynaecological Abnormalities

The reproductive tract, genital organs, develops from a system of embryonic ducts. These are the Müllerian and Wolffian ducts. In the female the Müllerian ducts develop whilst the Wolffian ducts regress and become vestigial. In the male the opposite takes place, so that the female has vestigial remnants of the Wolffian ducts and the male has vestigial remnants of the Müllerian ducts. The urinary system is also developed from these ducts.

DEVELOPMENTAL DISORDERS

In the female the genital tract is formed by fusion of the Müllerian ducts. This occurs from above and downwards so that eventually single cavities of the uterus and the vagina will be obvious. Fusion does not take place proximally so that two uterine (Fallopian) tubes develop from the unfused ends of the Müllerian ducts. If fusion fails to take place duplication of the uterus or vagina occur. The gonads develop differently. If the chromosomal pattern is normal the ovaries develop from a structure called coelomic epithelium which forms the urogenic ridge, from which the ovaries descend from their lumbar position into the pelvis. A structure called the *gubernaculum* contracts at this time and remains in life as the ovarian and round ligaments.

Uterine and vaginal defects

There are many variations in the type of uterine and vaginal defects, which can range from atresia to the combinations shown in figures 4.1 and 4.2.

UTERINE DIDELPHYS

During formation, fusion of the Müllerian ducts does not take place resulting in uterine didelphys or a double uterus (Fig. 4.1a). This means there are two uteri each with two uterine tubes, two cervices and two vaginae. Often slight fusion can be seen, but fundamentally the organs remain separate.

BICORNUATE UTERUS

With a bicornuate uterus (Fig. 4.1b) some fusion of the Müllerian ducts takes place but the uterus, cervix and vagina may be partially separated by a septum. This partial separation creates two horns of the uterus.

UNICORNUATE UTERUS

Maldevelopment of the Müllerian duct leads to the formation of a rudimentary asymmetrical horn on one side of the uterus, a unicornuate uterus (Fig. 4.1c).

34

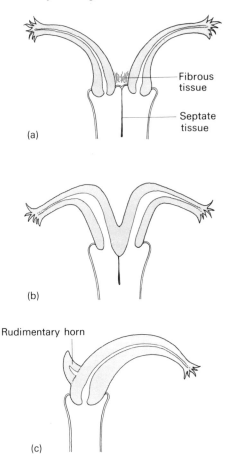

Fig. 4.1. Uterine defects: uterine didelphys (a), bicornuate uterus (b), unicornuate uterus (c).

SEPTATE UTERUS

A septate uterus (Fig. 4.2a) involves the septum projecting downwards in the uterine cavity to varying degrees. Usually the uterus, cervix and vagina are divided.

SUBSEPTATE UTERUS

The septum of a subseptate uterus (Fig. 4.2b) exists only in the upper part of the uterus and may project at different angles.

These are but a few examples of malformations of the uterus, others do exist but are comparatively rare. The most common uterine malformations are septate, subseptate and bicornuate uterus. There can be complete atresia of the

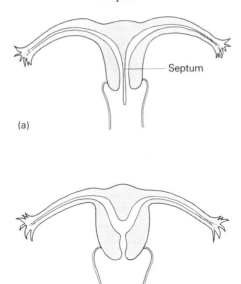

Septum

(a)

(b)

Fig. 4.2. Septum defects in the uterus: septate uterus (a), subseptate uterus (b).

uterus when only a fibrous nodule exists. A uterus may fail to develop and be found on examination to be infantile, perhaps due to agenesis of the ovaries and subsequent absence of female hormones which develop the sex organs.

CLINICAL FEATURES

Clinical features of these malformations may not be evident initially; they may be detected during a routine gynaecological examination. Occasionally however in the case of a septate vagina, dyspareunia and postcoital bleeding may occur. *Menorrhagia*, an excessive regular menstrual flow, may be caused by a double uterus since there is a greater endometrial area. *Recurrent abortion* is distressing and may be caused by double or subseptate uterus. Premature labour may also be a problem. An *ectopic pregnancy* may be found in the rudimentary horn of a uterus.

TREATMENT

Treatment will be given according to the symptoms or signs with which the patient presents.

In the case of an infantile (underdeveloped) uterus, oestrogen and progesterone preparations may be given by a doctor as therapeutic tests. When these drugs which are given orally are discontinued, withdrawal bleeding, should it occur, will be taken as a positive response.

Occasionally a double cavity uterus may be made single surgically. A vaginal septum may be divided surgically if dyspareunia is present.

Failure of canalization of the entry to the vagina can be found on examination at birth but more often it is found at puberty when the menarche has commenced but no menstrual flow is seen because the membrane behind the hymen has no perforation (*imperforate hymen*). The condition of menstrual fluid collecting in the vagina is called *cryptomenorrhoea*. As blood collects each month and builds up behind the hymen a definite bulge can be seen (Fig. 4.3). If this condition is unrelieved a back flow occurs leading to a condition of *haematocolpos* and eventually *haematosalpinx*. It is necessary for the haematocolpos to be drained (Fig. 4.4). The treatment and nursing care are dealt with in chapter 6.

Intersexuality

A discrepancy between various components of sexual manifestations: chromosomes, genitalia, hormones, or gender role, is an intersexual condition (Fream 1979).

Genetic sex determination

The nucleus of each body cell contains 46 chromosomes, 44 autosomes and 2 sex

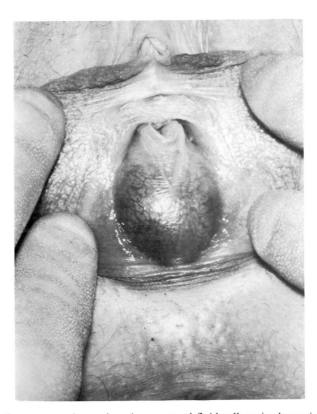

Fig. 4.3. Cryptomenorrhoea when the menstrual fluid collects in the vagina.

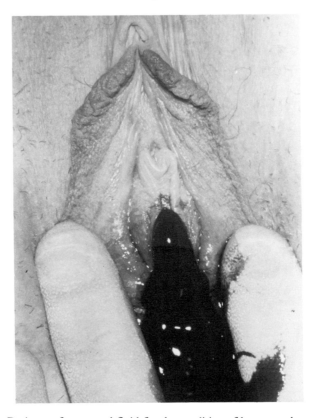

Fig. 4.4.   Drainage of menstrual fluid for the condition of haematocolpos.

chromosomes. When each cell divides the chromosomes duplicate themselves thereby producing two daughter cells containing 46 chromosomes, this process of cell division is called *mitosis.*

In *meiosis* which is a reduction division of the reproductive cells the oöcytes and spermatozoa (gametes) have their number of chromosomes reduced from 46 to 23 that is from being diploid (double) they become haploid (half) (Fig. 4.5). When fertilization takes place the oöcyte and spermatozoon each donate their 23 chromosomes and become diploid in number again—this then is referred to as the fertilized ovum.

In the normal female the sex chromosomes are XX, in the normal male XY. When the gametes, the oöcytes and the spermatozoa, are formed, all oöcytes carry the X chromosome and half the spermatozoa carry the X and the other half the Y. The resulting offspring are either XX, female or XY, male. It is the Y chromosome which dictates whether the body organization is male or female.

Most sex chromosome abnormalities arise from nondisjunction, that is, the pair of sex chromosomes (XX) fail to separate during meiosis. This may mean the oöcyte contains two X chromosomes or none. Fertilization by a spermatozoon which may carry a X or Y will result in abnormal patterns: XXX,

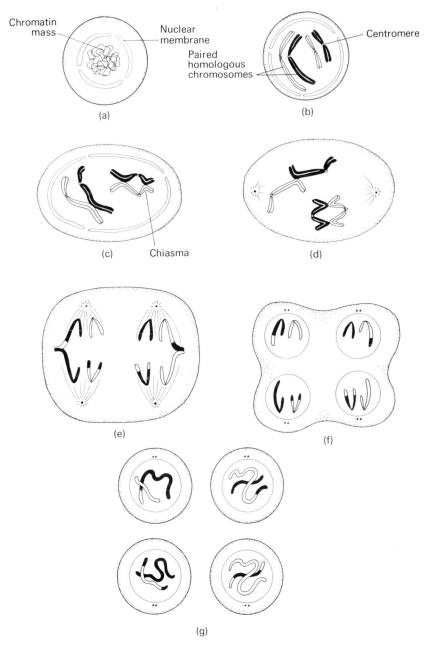

Chromatin mass

Nuclear membrane

Paired homologous chromosomes

Centromere

(a)

(b)

(c) Chiasma

(d)

(e)

(f)

(g)

Fig. 4.5. Meiosis: chromatin masses in the centre (a), chromosomes appear and homologous chromosomes pair and duplicate (b). Material is exchanged at the chiasmata (c), and homologous chromosomes move to opposite ends (d). The chromatids then separate (e) and four nuclei appear, each enclosing the haploid number of chromosomes (f). The cytoplasm then divides to form four gametes (g).

XXY or XO. YO must be incompatible with life for there is no known record of this aberration.

HERMAPHRODITISM, OR GONADAL INTERSEX

An individual who has mixed gonads, i.e., mixed intersex with testicular and ovarian tissue, is a true hermaphrodite, which is rare. The abnormality more likely to be seen is either *female hermaphroditism* in which intersex is of ovarian tissue, but external characteristics may be ambiguous, or *male hermaphroditism* in which intersex is of testicular tissue but external characteristics are ambiguous. Since these are not mixed intersex the outcome is not true hermaphroditism but *pseudohermaphroditism*, the patient having specific gonads but displaying the opposite external genitalia, or genitalia which appears ambiguous.

TURNER'S SYNDROME, OR GONADAL DYSGENESIS

In Turner's syndrome, the phenotype (body type) is female but the ovaries are represented as streaks of fibrous tissue. Because the ovaries are rudimentary, secondary sex characteristics do not develop such as breasts, development and distribution of axillary and pubic hair. Menstruation does not occur.

This is an abnormality brought about by a chromosome deficiency. The chromosome combination or *karyotype* is usually 45 XO. It can be seen that a second X chromosome is absent; in a normal female the karyotype would be 46 XX.

Other common features of Turner's syndrome are a shortness of stature, and webbing of the neck. The woman is amenorrhoeic and infertile.

KLINEFELTER'S SYNDROME

Klinefelter's syndrome is also a chromosomal abnormality. The karyotype is 47 XXY. Here there is an extra female chromosome although the phenotype of the individual is male, very tall with normal external genitalia. Other features are a high pitched feminine voice, rather effeminate clear skin and adipose tissue deposits, e.g., gynaecomastia. These patients are also infertile, and this condition may be associated with mental defects.

ANDROGEN OVERSECRETION ANOMALIES

Production of cortisol is affected if there is a deficiency in an enzyme (C21 hydroxylase) in the adrenal gland. If cortisol is not produced or produced in insufficient amounts the amount of adrenocorticotrophic hormone (ACTH) is increased. When this occurs excessive amounts of androgens are circulating which causes developmental anomalies of the external genitalia. In females, the androgens affect the labia which fuses together, the clitoris enlarges and the genitalia takes on a masculine form rather like hypospadias. In males, in the presence of excessive amounts of circulating androgens there is a correspondingly excessive masculine growth hence the term 'Infant Hercules'. Early sexual functioning is evident also.

TESTICULAR FEMINIZATION

With testicular feminization the karyotype is 46 XY. Androgens are secreted but the tissues are apparently insensitive and the phenotype develops along female lines. This patient may present at a gynaecological outpatients department complaining of amenorrhoea. On examination there may be a very short vagina and the uterus absent. The gonads in this case are testes which remain in the abdomen, or are found on examination to be in the labia. The testicles may undergo malignant change and should be removed at puberty.

GENDER ROLE

Gender role or psychological sex is usually developed in accordance with the phenotype, i.e., genital sex. Occasionally environmental factors and close profound relationships may significantly affect the psychological sex of an individual. It is arguable whether homosexuality has a chromosomal entity, but work on this theory is inconclusive. Although it has been shown recently that basic sexual differentiation is determined by genes, it may be that further work will reveal more definite correlation between gonads and psychological abnormalities. Whatever gender role the individual displays, sympathetic understanding and tolerance from society in general are essential if great unhappiness is to be avoided.

Management of intersex conditions

Full investigation is essential which includes thorough physical examination and full laboratory investigation. Even then sex diagnosis may be inconclusive.

BARR BODIES

Barr bodies or sex chromatins are found by examining material obtained from a buccal smear. In genetic females a Barr body, which is a small mass of chromatin, is found on the nuclear membrane (Fig. 4.6). This establishes that there is XX karyotype. The absence of a barr body usually indicates that an individual is male, i.e., XY chromosomes, but the karyotype XO would not be detected by the simple absence of a barr body.

BLOOD INVESTIGATIONS

Another way of determining sex from nuclear analysis is the presence of a *drumstick* on the polymorphonuclear leucocytes in the genetic female (Fig. 4.7). Other

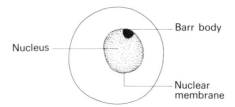

Fig. 4.6.   Barr body or sex chromatin within the nucleus of a genetic female cell.

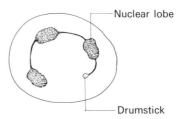

Fig. 4.7.   Drumstick-like mass attached to one of the nuclear lobes in polymorpho-nuclear leucocytes in genetic females.

investigations may include laparoscopic examination under general anaesthesia and hormone assays. The aim of arriving at a correct diagnosis is to make sure that a child is reared in the correct sex.

Treatment

Treatment includes surgical excision of any redundant genitalia, or surgical modification which the patient requests or finds acceptable. The type of surgery performed will depend very much upon the gender role and may include clitori-dectomy and vaginoplasty. If the gender role is male then mastectomy and closure of a hypospadias may be undertaken. Hormones may be given to develop sexual organs, especially the breast in Turner's syndrome. Suppression of ACTH in androgen oversecretion may be useful.

Whatever the treatment psychological support at all times is absolutely essential.

This chapter is simply a brief introduction to some of the conditions of inter-sex, works which cover this subject fully can be found in the references and further reading.

5 Menstruation

Menstruation, unless it is precocious, usually begins at puberty between the ages of 11 and 14. It is the regular discharge of blood, mucus and tissue debris from the uterus at regular intervals.

THE MENSTRUAL CYCLE

Menstruation is described as having a cycle which may be very variable but is generally considered normal if it occurs every 28 days. The actual time of bleeding is between 4 and 7 days, but again is variable. The actual amount of blood loss is approximately 50 ml to 200 ml at each monthly menstruation.

Control of menstruation begins in the cerebral cortex of the brain which influences the hypothalamus, which in turn influences the anterior lobe of the pituitary gland (Fig. 5.1). The hypothalamus stimulates the anterior lobe of the pituitary gland to produce follicle stimulating hormone (FSH), luteinizing hormone (LH) and prolactin. These are called the *gonadatrophic* hormones since their target organ is the female gonad, i.e., the ovary.

The pituitary gland responds to levels of oestrogen and progesterone in the circulating bloodstream. If the blood level of oestrogen is low the pituitary gland responds by producing FSH; if the blood level of oestrogen is high then the production of FSH is inhibited. This mechanism is called a *negative feedback control* and is shown more clearly in diagrammatic form (Fig. 5.2). The same effect is produced in relationship to blood levels of progesterone.

The plus factor or positive feedback mechanism of oestrogen is explained by the fact that the corpus luteum as well as producing progesterone also produces a small amount of oestrogen after ovulation and this prevents the endometrium from breaking down prematurely.

The blood levels of progesterone and oestrogen vary during menstruation (Fig. 5.3a), during pregnancy (Fig. 5.3b) and during the years of the menopause (Fig. 5.3c).

SUMMARY

The menstrual cycle can be tabulated thus:

1 The hypothalamus acts upon the anterior lobe of the pituitary gland stimulating it to produce the gonadatrophic hormones.

2 These are follicle stimulating hormone FSH, luteinizing hormone LH and prolactin (which stimulates lactation).

3 The FSH acts upon the ovary resulting in the maturation of a primary, or primordial, follicle. This is a primitive ovum surrounded by a single layer of epithelial cells.

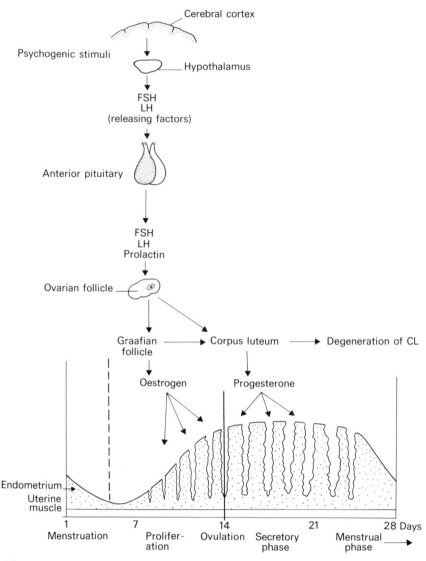

Fig. 5.1. The physiology of menstruation.

4 The primary follicle becomes the *Graafian follicle* which gradually ripens and becomes distended.

5 At this point oestrogen is being produced by the Graafian follicle, this acts on the endometrial lining of the uterus, producing repair and regrowth. This is the *proliferative* phase.

6 The Graafian follicle then approaches the under surface of the ovary, bulges and gently ruptures releasing its ovum (*ovulation*).

7 The luteinizing hormone now stimulates the growth of the corpus luteum

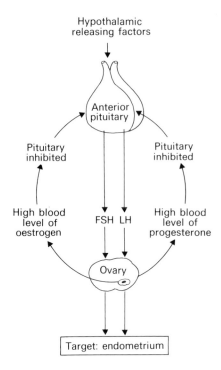

Fig. 5.2. The negative feedback mechanism of progesterone and oestrogen levels in the blood.

and causes it to produce progesterone. This hormone also acts on the endometrial lining of the uterus and produces changes in the deep endometrium. Glands in the endometrium now become more highly developed and active, they produce glycogen and mucus, and other nutrients which would be available if fertilization took place. This phase of the menstrual cycle is the *secretory* phase.

8 If the ovum is not fertilized by a sperm there is a sudden fall in the blood levels of progesterone and oestrogen due to the degeneration of the corpus luteum.

9 The endometrium now begins to degenerate; cells and glandular tissue, deprived of progesterone and oestrogen, die and bleeding begins. The endometrium regresses down to the basal layer.

10 The cycle now begins again and the endometrium begins its regenerative process.

Hormones

DURING PREGNANCY

If fertilization of the ovum takes place the normal menstrual cycle is interrupted. Once the placenta begins its development from the trophoblast it is capable of

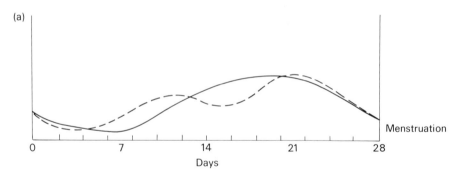

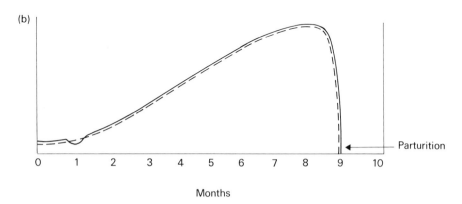

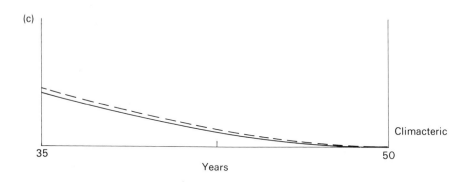

Fig. 5.3. Blood levels of progesterone (solid line) and oestrogen (hatched line) during different cycles of a woman's life: menstruation (a), pregnancy (b), menopause (c).

hormone production. This hormone is the *chorionic gonadatrophin* and like the luteinizing hormone maintains the function of the corpus luteum. As the pregnancy progresses more of the hormonal function is taken over by the placenta, eventually at about the twelfth week of pregnancy the corpus luteum degenerates and the placenta secretes increasing amounts of oestrogen and progesterone, until full term is reached.

Summary

Hormones in pregnancy may be summarized thus:
1 Fertilization takes place and the corpus luteum and its function is maintained by the luteinizing hormone.
2 The developing embryo forms a trophoblast which secretes chorionic gonadatrophin.
3 The chorionic gonadatrophin helps to maintain the corpus luteum, and its continued production of progesterone.
4 As the trophoblast develops it becomes the *placenta* and by the twelfth week the corpus luteum has degenerated and both oestrogen and progesterone are produced more than adequately by the placenta.
5 This extra oestrogen and progesterone output is necessary for growth and development of the lactiferous glands and ducts of the breast.
6 After delivery, or parturition, the blood levels of both oestrogen and progesterone fall dramatically and the pituitary gland is able to secrete FSH to begin the menstrual cycle again.

POSTNATALLY

A return to normal menstrual cycle may be delayed and a period of amenorrhoea experienced by mothers who are breastfeeding their babies. This is probably because the suckling reflex causes an excessive secretion of prolactin which in turn inhibits the pituitary gland's production of FSH, and subsequently inhibits production of the Graafian follicle and thus the normal cycle.

DURING DEVELOPMENT

Pituitary and ovarian function varies with each phase of a woman's life. At birth the ovaries of a female child contain up to 200,000 primary, or primordial follicles which remain undeveloped up until the child is about 7 or 8 years old. Then a few years before puberty the gonadatrophic hormones increase sufficiently to promote primary follicle development. This indicates that the hypothalamus and pituitary glands are maturing gradually and producing their FSH- and LH-releasing factors. This may be referred to as the prepubertal stage of the child's development.

PUBERTY

At puberty around the ages of 11 to 15 years many of the primary follicles are producing oestrogen and just one of these follicles undergoes further maturation to become the Graafian follicle (see Fig. 5.1). At this stage oestrogen is promoting the development of breast tissue and is partly responsible for changes in the outline and contour of the body. The girl is now ready to move into her reproductive phase of life and experience her first menstrual period, the menarche. The acceleration of oestrogen secretion which occurs produces the menarche. Vaginal glycogen content is increased and there may be an obvious vaginal discharge. The pH of the vagina is altered from alkaline to acid. Axillary and pubic hair are evident.

Emotional aspects

Puberty can be and often is a difficult transitional stage to go through. Some girls may feel rather sensitive and shy about their new shape and extra features. It is at this time that a girl might experience a tremendously increased awareness of herself and her body and its function which may lead to emotional upheaval. Tact and understanding are essential when dealing with such a girl. Bewilderment and anxiety may be experienced if timely and sensible explanations of this process of development are not adequately explained. Adolescence, or 'youth', includes the period of puberty and extends to maturity. It is vital that proper preparation for adolescence is made early on in life so that emotional upheaval can be avoided or eased.

Schools play a major part in this preparation but parental influence is probably more valuable if approached in the right way at the right time. Frank and open discussions on sexual development and sexual activity will dispel much of the uncertainty and anxiety that is felt by adolescents on these issues. Some parents, however, may not approach these discussions with equanimity and some adolescents may feel unable to approach their parents; the teenager must be given access to literature or counsellors on these issues. The adolescent girl may be frequently encountered on a gynaecological ward and the nurse must be aware of the problems ignorance might create. Often the nurse will be young and herself experiencing many of her patient's developmental problems, this though can be put to good use and provide a sound basis for understanding.

THE MENOPAUSE

Menopause, the other end of the scale in the menstrual cycle, is another transitional phase of a woman's life which can be achieved relatively smoothly with the only obvious manifestation being a cessation of menstruation, or it may be a physically and psychologically difficult time of life. In fact many women may dread the approach of the menopause and just as in puberty the realization of approaching sexuality causes some trepidation so too does the menopause with the reproductive phase of life over. This may involve a preconception of loss of femininity, loss of libido and a definite feeling of having embarked upon middle age with a vengeance. Exaggerated stories exchanged in various social situations do nothing to dispel apprehension.

Nurse's role

The nurse will be able to help women develop an informed approach to the menopause by counselling them. The menopause usually occurs in one of the following ways:

1 Menstruation may stop abruptly and not return.
2 The intervals between menstruation lengthen.
3 The blood loss at menstruation gradually diminishes.
4 Menstruation becomes irregular and unpredictable.

Advice should include details about diet and exercise to help the patient retain or possibly improve her body shape and minimize hot flushes precipitated by spicy foods. Also included would be guidelines for maintaining a state of good general health.

The nurse can help the patient by promoting an optimistic attitude to the menopause by educating and reassuring her about the symptoms. The cessation of menstruation is caused by a lowered oestrogen output and it is this lowering of oestrogen (and progesterone) output which produces the physical changes experienced at this time. When ovarian function has ceased it is called the climacteric but generally the term *menopause* is used to indicate the end of the reproductive phase. More correctly reproduction stops a year or two earlier with anovular cycles.

Recommending relevant literature may also be helpful. Books such as *The Menopause, A Positive Attitude* by Rosetta Reitz and *The Menopause* by Mary Anderson help women to anticipate and deal positively with psychological and physical changes. Positive factors which a nurse should refer to are: relief from monthly menstruation and freedom from unwanted pregnancies.

CLINICAL FEATURES

Hot flushes

The most common symptoms of the menopause which can be particularly distressing to a woman are hot flushes. They are caused by vasomotor dilation producing a wave of heat with a red flush spreading from the neck to the face. They may occur 5-6 times an hour or once or twice a day. Profuse sweating may accompany these flushes and bedclothing may be saturated at night; because a chill follows the hot flush the woman may be constantly putting on or taking off her jacket. Alcohol or hot foods may aggravate or precipitate a hot flush. Hot flushes are clearly a social inconvenience to many women.

Somatic alterations

The classical 'middle age' spread may manifest itself with fat depositions in the breasts, buttocks and abdominal regions. It may be due to overeating as a compensatory mechanism to cope with depression which may occur at this time of life.

Diminishing muscle control is caused by decreased circulating oestrogen and leads to postural changes. Hair growth may appear around the mouth and chin. Other body changes, e.g., osteoarthritis, osteoporosis, may be noticed and are caused by the withdrawal of oestrogen affecting calcium metabolism. There may be a slight reduction in height because of calcium deficiency.

Organic changes

There is a general regression of the genital organs. The vulva and vagina undergo very gradual atrophy, the uterus and appendages also become reduced in size. Again because of the withdrawal of oestrogen the pH of the vagina is altered and infections more likely. Sexual intercourse may become difficult because of a loss of elasticity of vaginal tissue.

Other changes

Gastrointestinal upsets may cause constipation, dyspepsia and excessive flatulence. Pelvic ligaments may become relaxed and not as supportive allowing prolapse of the pelvic organs. This may lead to urinary incontinence (see chap. 8). Some authorities cite the effects of oestrogen deficiency around the time of the menopause as a cause of incontinence, frequency or dysuria. Oestrogen deficiency may affect the mucosa of the urethra and bladder causing these urinary disturbances, but stress and anxiety at this time may affect urinary control. A certain nervous tension may be experienced leading to irritability and emotional outbursts.

Treatment

It is *abnormal* for bleeding to be profuse or prolonged, and it is important that such signs be investigated. Before the menopause is achieved, some 25% of women seek help. Help can be readily available in the form of sympathetic understanding from family and friends. Tolerant attitudes are essential toward unpredictable mood swings and emotional outbursts. It can be a difficult time for all the family as at this time children are experiencing the problems associated with adolescence. The medical help sought at this time can provide the necessary explanation of the physical and psychological upheavals being experienced.

Cosmetic advice will be appreciated. Creams are available which will remove unwanted facial hair and moisturising creams may be suggested, all with a view to providing a morale boost from an improved appearance.

Tranquillizers may have a place in treating 'nerves' or depression and it is now felt that women need not expect a dismissive attitude from their doctors towards their menopausal symptoms. Since most symptoms of the menopause are due to oestrogen deficiency, if they become troublesome they can be treated by hormone replacement therapy (HRT). Considerable controversy exists regarding HRT as it is known that breast and genital malignancies are supported by oestrogen; it would therefore be unwise to encourage HRT in these circumstances. Replacement therapy can be of value it its effects are monitored, adjusted and it is prescribed by doctor. The symptom most easily treated by oestrogen replacement is the hot flush.

The use of cyclical HRT to preserve youth or to prevent 'growing old' is potentially dangerous, very debatable, and the subject of much research. If the menopause has been artificially induced by bilateral removal of the ovaries, HRT may be needed as the symptoms may be sudden and rather severe. Oestrogen may be given orally as Ethinyloestradiol 10-50 μg daily, or as a single subdermal pellet usually implanted in the abdominal wall. These 'implants' may be effective for 3-6 months and can be renewed in the outpatient clinic.

REPLACEMENT THERAPY

Postmenopausal oestrogen replacement is particularly controversial because of the risk of endometrial cancer and other diseases. Benefits of oestrogen replacement therapy may involve the improvement or retardation of:
1 Vasomotor symptoms.
2 Atrophic genitourinary changes.
3 Osteoporosis.
4 Cardiovascular disease (atherosclerosis).
5 Sleep disturbance or depression.
   The risks may include:
1 Endometrial neoplasia.
2 Breast neoplasia.
3 Thromboembolism.
4 Hypertension.
   The major question still to be answered is, do the benefits outweigh the risks. Research may eventually clear much of the controversy.

DISORDERS OF MENSTRUATION

Amenorrhoea, dysfunctional uterine bleeding, menorrhagia, metropathia haemorrhagica, intermenstrual bleeding, and postmenopausal bleeding are all disorders of menstruation. Other names used to classify these disorders are: epimenorrhoea, polymenorrhoea and hypermenorrhoea. These terms all mean excessive vaginal bleeding but are used less often. Conversely hypomenorrhoea and oligomenorrhoea are used occasionally to describe scanty or infrequent periods.

Amenorrhoea

Amenorrhoea is defined as an absence of menstrual periods and can be classified as false, physiological or pathological in origin (Fig. 5.4). False amenorrhoea is when menstruation is occurring but is concealed, i.e., cryptomenorrhoea (see

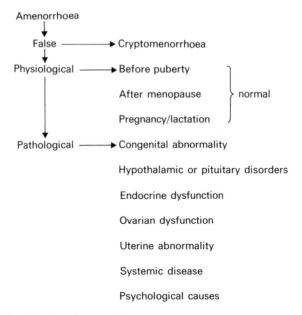

Fig. 5.4.   Classification of amenorrhoea.

chap. 4). Amenorrhoea exists if the uterus is surgically removed, or the ovaries are removed or destroyed, e.g., by irradiation.

If menstruation has never occurred amenorrhoea is said to be *primary. Secondary* amenorrhoea exists when a normal menstrual pattern had been established but since ceased.

A complete classification is difficult and I acknowledge that this is by no means complete. What it serves to do is to represent the wide range of distressing symptoms which the patient suffers. Depression and emotional upheaval naturally accompanies many of the conditions which cause amenorrhoea; the nurse must remember that amenorrhoea is a *symptom* of disease and not a disease in itself.

Thorough investigation is required to determine the cause before treatment is instigated. Physical examination is essential and should breast changes be evident, pregnancy should be excluded as this is the *most common* cause of amenorrhoea (in the reproductive era). Oral contraceptives are occasionally responsible for secondary amenorrhoea, this happens if the pill has caused endometrial atrophy.

CLASSIFICATION OF PATHOLOGICAL AMENORRHOEA

Amenorrhoea can be *one* of the symptoms of a disorder and these patients may not necessarily be treated by gynaecologist. Endocrine disorders (see Table 5.1) and particularly pituitary causes of amenorrhoea are rare but would fall into this category.

Table 5.1 Endocrine causes of pathological amenorrhoea.

Organ	Clinical signs
Hypothalamus	Fröhlich's syndrome (dystrophia adiposogenitalis): hirsutism, obesity, lethargy, mental dullness, genital hypoplasia.
Pituitary	Chiari-Frommel syndrome: persistent galactorrhoea with suppression of FSH and LH production. Sheehan's syndrome (Simmonds' disease): pituitary atrophy, genital atrophy, sterility, loss of libido.
Thyroid	Hypothyroidism or hyperthyroidism: symptoms of thyroid disturbance with amenorrhoea.
Adrenal	Addison's disease (adrenal failure): metabolic disturbance, gonadotrophic depression. Cushing's syndrome (adrenal hyperplasia): overactivity of the adrenal gland, increased secretion of androgens resulting in masculinization, hirsutism and muscularity.
Ovaries	Arrhenoblastoma, agenesis: masculinizing effects, deepening of the voice, atrophy or the breast and hypertrophy of the clitoris. Stein-Leventhal syndrome (polycystic ovaries): hirsutism, infertility and amenorrhoea.

Congenital

With congenital amenorrhoea there will be hypoplasia of the uterus or ovaries or gonadal dysgenesis. It may also be due to chromosomal abnormalities (see chap.4).

Systemic disease

Systemic and debilitating disease, e.g., tuberculosis, renal disease, and malnutrition may all cause amenorrhoea. Psychiatric disorders may also be the cause.

Psychological disturbances

Environmental changes may produce stress and subsequently amenorrhoea. Bereavement, grief, emotional disturbance, and obesity, which may be a result of a depressive illness, may cause amenorrhoea. It is common for young women suffering from anorexia nervosa to experience amenorrhoea.

INVESTIGATIONS

The gynaecologist will avoid an unnecessary battery of tests if he or she thinks that the amenorrhoea may be transient and due to emotional disturbance of some kind. Tests are also usually avoided until the patient reaches the age of 17 in the case of primary amenorrhoea or if a pregnancy is desired in a woman with secondary amenorrhoea.

A pregnancy test is the first test to rule out the commonest cause of secondary amenorrhoea. Then possibly further investigations will be carried out:

1 Full general examination including a pelvic examination.
2 Blood investigations for evidence of infection or anaemia.
3 Chest X-ray to rule out tuberculosis.
4 Skull X-rays to exclude pituitary tumours.
5 Vaginal cytology to reveal oestrogen presence.
6 Urine assays for 24-hours to estimate hormonal levels.
7 Chromosomal analysis to exclude chromosomal abnormalities.

Specific

More specific investigations will include an endometrial and ovarian biopsy, a laparoscopy and hysterosalpingography.

NURSE'S ROLE

During all of these examinations adequate support and reassurance will be needed. An adolescent may feel that she is abnormal as most of her peers will be menstruating regularly. A married woman who is being investigated for second-ary amenorrhoea and is anxious to start her family may be experiencing guilt feelings and matrimonial discord. As for the woman whose amenorrhoea is a symptom of a pituitary or hypothalamic disorder she may be very concerned about her body image and distressed about her hirsutism and possible masculine appearance. Nurses aware of the patient's potential reactions to these problems will be able to plan nursing care with all the insight required and thus, having identified potential problems, help the patient to cope with and overcome them over a period of time.

TREATMENT

Treatment will be based on any systemic disease which may be responsible or any endocrine or psychiatric disorder which has been found to be the cause of amenorrhoea. Antibiotic therapy may be prescribed for an infection and iron replacement therapy for anaemia may correct amenorrhoea. Hormone therapy may be given to induce menstruation and drugs, e.g., clomiphine (Clomid), may be tried in the hope of stimulating ovulation. Advice on diet in obesity and anorexia may be helpful.

Occasionally surgical treatment may be tried if the amenorrhoea is caused by polycystic ovaries (Stein-Leventhal syndrome). Wedge resection of both ovaries is often successful in restoring ovulation and menstruation.

Psychological support throughout is essential with explanations and options presented to the patient, and her husband if she is married, as cooperation from all concerned is required if results are to be successful.

Dysfunctional uterine bleeding

Uterine bleeding for which no precise cause is discovered is referred to as dysfunctional uterine bleeding (DUB). Menorrhagia and metropathia haemorrhagica may both be included under DUB as quite often no cause can be found for either. Emotional disturbances and strain are often implicated as causes of amenorrhoea. Dysfunctional uterine bleeding has been defined as 'the occurrence of irregular or excessive bleeding from the uterus in the absence of pregnancy, infection, trauma, new growth or hormone treatment' (Barnes 1983).

Menorrhagia

Heavy or profuse menstrual bleeding usually occurring at regular intervals is referred to as menorrhagia. Clots may be passed which suggests that the anticlotting mechanism of the uterus cannot cope with the excessive blood flow. In general, menorrhagia is caused by a pathological condition, which increases the size of the endometrium. Other possible causes are: uterine fibromyomata, cervical erosion or polyp, carcinoma of the cervix or body of the uterus, salpingooöphoritis, endometriosis, pelvic inflammatory disease, cystic ovaries, and a retroverted or prolapsed uterus. In addition, anaemia or blood dyscrasia, e.g., thrombocytopenia, may be the cause. Just as amenorrhoea may be caused by hypothalamic or pituitary disorders so may menorrhagia; hormonal imbalance similarly may cause amenorrhoea or menorrhagia.

Metropathia haemorrhagica

A disorder which does not exhibit any obvious physical signs or symptoms is metropathia haemorrhagica. It is perhaps the best example of dysfunctional bleeding. Hormonal imbalance, in particular excessive production of oestrogen without progesterone, produces hyperplasia of the endometrium. When this tissue is examined microscopically it is seen to be glandular and cystic. It rather resembles 'Swiss cheese' and its full title is cystic glandular hyperplasia of the endometrium.

Intermenstrual bleeding

The term intermenstrual is literal and denotes uterine bleeding *in between* menstrual periods. The amount of bleeding is slight and may not be menstrual bleeding at all. It may confuse the patient so that she may not be able to calculate her cycle accurately. The causes may include cervical erosions and polyps or malignant disease of the uterus.

Postmenopausal bleeding

Probably the most sinister type of uterine bleeding is postmenopausal (PMB) as it must always be regarded as a *possible* sign of genital malignancy. It may indicate malignancy or a benign tumour, i.e., a cervical polyp. An infection may also cause bleeding. Bleeding is considered to be postmenopausal when it occurs a year or more after the completion of the menopause. Whenever this does occur it must be treated with the utmost gravity and must be investigated promptly.

INVESTIGATIONS

A thorough general and pelvic examination is always done and a detailed history taken. The patient's environmental and social circumstances must be carefully noted as they may well have a bearing on her condition. Precise details of the menstrual cycle will help in arriving at the correct diagnosis. If further tests are to be undertaken, the nurse will have to prepare the patient for special diagnostic investigations. These may include:

1 Vaginal and cervical cytology.
2 Blood investigations, e.g., a full blood count and haemoglobin estimate, bleeding and coagulation times, oestrogen, progesterone and prolactin studies, and a FSH and LH assay.
3 Examination under anaesthetic with laparoscopy, colposcopy or hysteroscopy.
4 Curettage which will be diagnostic and may reveal an intrauterine lesion, e.g., tuberculosis or carcinoma.
5 Hormonal studies, i.e., urinary gonadotrophins.
6 Ultrasound scan.

TREATMENT

Treatment will be based on treating the cause if this is detected, the age of the patient, and the desire for children. In women under 40 treatment is usually conservative whilst in women over 40 treatment may be surgical. Correction of an iron deficiency anaemia, however, will be essential whatever the age of the woman.

Hormone therapy

Hormones will only be prescribed when a thorough examination and investigation have been done and a pregnancy is desired. The danger otherwise would be the masking of a malignant disease. Oestrogen-only preparations are best avoided because they naturally cause proliferation of the endometrium. Combination therapy with oestrogen and progesterone is usually effective, e.g., the contraceptive pill, Controvlar, which contains norethisterone acetate 3 mg and ethinyloestradiol 50 μg. A progestogen preparation used is norethisterone (Primolut N) taken orally, 15 mg to 30 mg daily, can be effective in controlling heavy bleeding.

Surgery

Curettage involving the removal of the surface layer of endometrium is essentially a diagnostic procedure but it may be of some therapeutic value if only temporarily. Hysterectomy, removal of the uterus, will be necessary in women over 40 who do not respond to other forms of treatment, or for whom hormone therapy would be contraindicated.

General

The patient should be advised to take adequate rest during a heavy period. It may be advisable for her to rest in bed if uterine haemorrhage is severe. Occasionally adjustments in life-style may be approprate, and with the help of the family she should try to avoid physical and mental stress. If necessary a tranquillizer may be prescribed.

6 The Vulva and Vagina

ANATOMY OF THE VULVA

The *vulva* is the collective name given to the external genitalia. It comprises: the mons pubis, labia majora and minora, clitoris, perineum, hymen, and bulbs of the vestibule (Fig. 6.1).

The mons pubis (mons veneris)

The *mons pubis* or *mons veneris* is a triangular structure with a horizontal upper border. It is a protective pad of adipose tissue overlying the symphysis pubis and is covered by skin containing sweat glands. At puberty a growth of hair will cover the mons pubis. The mons pubis affords a cushioning effect during coitus.

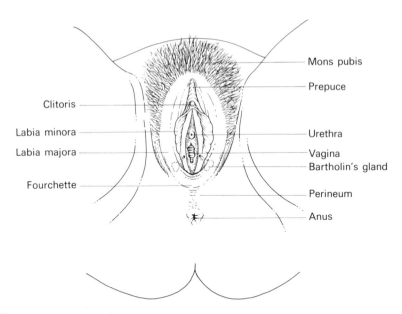

Fig. 6.1. Anatomy of the vulva.

Labia majora

The *labia majora* are longitudinal folds of flesh which form the lateral boundaries of the vulva. They extend from the mons pubis anteriorly to the perineum posteriorly. They comprise of adipose tissue covered by skin and contain a number of sebaceous glands. Their outer surfaces are covered by hair, their inner surfaces are smooth.

The function of the labia majora is protective. The adipose tissue has a cushioning effect, and the folds guard the entrance to the vagina.

The Bartholin's glands, or vestibular glands lie in the deeper parts of the posterior one third of the labia majora and the ducts open into the vaginal orifice providing a mucus lubrication during sexual intercourse. Although only pea sized, the Bartholin's glands can frequently become infected.

Labia minora

The *labia minora*, as the name suggests, are smaller folds of flesh, also covered by skin but without the padding of adipose tissue, or hair. They lie within the labia majora and form a triangular area known as the vestibule. The apex of the triangle is the prepuce and the base is the fourchette.

These smaller folds are vascular and well-supplied with nerve endings. They become engorged and erectile when sexually stimulated. Protection is their function as they close over the entrance to the vagina. It is in the vestibule that urethral and vaginal orifices are found.

The clitoris

The *clitoris* is a small erectile structure which lies under the mons pubis protected by the prepuce which is the hooded structure at the apex of the triangular vestibule. It is well-supplied by nerve endings and is one of the main erogenous zones of the female. It is a vascular structure, which becomes engorged during sexual activity and is considered to be the female equivalent of the penis.

The perineum

The *perineum* lies between the fourchette and the anus and is covered by perineal skin and some hair. The perineal body is the underlying structure; this is a fibromuscular body which is the merging point of the levator ani and pelvic floor muscles.

The hymen

The *hymen* is a thin membrane which forms a diaphragm at the entrance to the vagina. It normally has one or more perforations. Its function is protective in the prepubertal period. Historically the hymen, if it remained intact, was considered to be proof of virginity but today modern sanitary aids such as tampons result in a torn hymen without coitus taking place. After childbirth the hymen is completely torn but tags still remain around the vaginal orifice; these are called carunculae myrtiformes, or hymenales.

Bulbs of the vestibule

Bulbs of the vestibule or *vestibular bulbs* are two elongated structures situated to either side of the vaginal orifice and composed of erectile tissue that is joined to the clitoris anteriorly. They lie under the labia minora. The Bartholin's glands are embedded in these structures.

The nerve supply to the vulva and perineum is via the pudendal nerve. The blood supply to the vulva and the venous drainage is via the internal and external pudendal vessels. Lymphatic drainage of the vulva is mainly to the superficial inguinal glands and then to deeper inguinal and femoral glands. This lymphatic drainage is of significance when considering surgical treatment for carcinoma of the vulva.

CONDITIONS OF THE VULVA

The vulva undergoes certain change in relation to the woman's age and during pregnancy. In pregnancy the vulva may become pigmented; in the reproductive phase of a woman's life the labia majora cover the labia minora whilst in prepuberty and menopausal women this is not so. This is because the vulva is not sufficiently developed prepuberty and then is deprived of oestrogen at the menopause and atrophies.

The classification of vulval conditions is complicated by the fact that whilst the patient may be referred to a gynaecologist both a dermatologist and a venereologist can be involved in the treatment. I shall describe the most common vulval conditions.

Pruritus vulvae

Pruritus vulvae, sometimes called itchy vulva, is extremely common. There are many causes which produce this intense itching, leading to an overwhelming desire to obtain relief by scratching the area.

So intense is the itching that I have known at least two patients who have confessed to sitting in a cold shallow bath for most of the night. Each episode of scratching is likely to produce tissue damage and thus aggravate the condition. Fatigue and warmth are liable to heighten the itching so that women with pruritus vulvae will suffer more at bedtime.

Many local applications may be self-prescribed but these will only make the condition much worse. Many women suffer with pruritus vulvae for years before they seek medical attention, by which time repeated trauma may have led to malignant changes taking place.

POSSIBLE CAUSES

Pruritus vulvae may be caused by vaginal discharge, poor vulval hygiene, toxic states, general diseases, skin conditions, carcinoma or psychological factors.

A vaginal discharge may be due to *Trichomonas vaginalis* or *Candida albicans*, or may increase during pregnancy or whilst taking the contraceptive pill. Poor vulval hygiene may contribute to pruritus. Toxic states can be caused by jaundice, Hodgkin's disease or uraemia. General diseases, e.g., diabetes (glycosuria), or a deficiency disease, e.g., iron deficiency, avitaminosis A and B, may lead to pruritus. Skin conditions affecting the vulva include:

Tinea, scabies, threadworm, herpes, intertrigo

Contact dermatitis—soaps, chemicals, contraceptive creams

Primary atrophy (*kraurosis*), lichen sclerosus

Leucoplakia—hypertrophic changes of the vulva

With carcinoma of the vulva pruritus may be the only symptom. Psychological causes may be brought about by sexual frustration, cancer phobia, or anxiety states. In psychological causes a vicious circle is set in motion, itching may begin as a response to cortical stimulation then as relief is sought by scratching, the epithelium of the vulva is damaged and further itching occurs.

INVESTIGATION

Full investigation of pruritus vulvae is essential so that appropriate treatment may be prescribed and relief obtained as soon as possible. The possibility of malignancy **must** be ruled out.

A detailed investigation would include:

1 A full medical examination with a history of the complaint. This should reveal details of frequency and duration of itching, and what, if anything has been used to relieve the condition. Allergies may be discovered at this point.

2 A full blood count.

3 Repeated examination of vaginal discharge. This should be carried out to exclude Trichomonas and *Candida albicans.*

4 Urinalysis and glucose tolerance test to exclude diabetes.

5 Gastric analysis to exclude achlorhydria.

6 Skin biopsy to exclude carcinoma.

7 Careful discussion with the patient to try to discover a possible underlying psychogenic cause.

TREATMENT

Treatment should never be commenced without the benefit of full examination as occasionally a malignant condition may be masked for months or possibly years. When a cause has been found the treatment will be specific to that cause. A great many patients with pruritus vulvae will be found to have *Trichomonas vaginalis* and the treatment will be with metronidazole.

Other principles of treatment include:

1 Strict attention to vulval hygiene.

2 Avoidance of irritant soaps or other cosmetics, especially sprays.

3 Avoidance of irritant clothing, especially synthetic fabrics and restrictive underclothing.
4 Prescription of night sedation to allow adequate rest and an interruption in scratching.
5 Application of hydrocortisone cream 1% locally. Cold applications often afford temporary relief. Oestrogen therapy may help a postmenopasual patient.
6 Antihistamines may be given for allergies.
7 Relief from anxiety—hospitalization is occasionally needed to provide an atmosphere free from too much stress.
8 Sympathetic counselling.

If pruritus vulvae persists despite all efforts the last resort may be a simple vulvectomy.

Bartholin's cyst and abscess

Two common conditions of the Bartholin's gland are the formation of a cyst or an abscess.

With a *Bartholin's cyst*, the patient may complain of a 'lump' in the vulva. The cyst occurs when the tiny Bartholin's gland becomes blocked usually as a result of infection of the gland, *bartholinitis*, which produces fibrosis within the gland or duct. In this condition the cyst may be painless but secretion from the gland will be blocked.

The cyst may become acutely infected with *Streptococci*, *Staphylococci* or *Gonococci* or other infecting organisms. An abscess is extremely painful and tender; it will look red and swollen and feels hot. Examination may be difficult because the area is very painful. A patient with a *Bartholin's abscess* often presents herself to an accident or emergency department because of pain. Once the diagnosis has been made the patient is transferred to a gynaecological ward. The nurse must observe existing hospital policy regarding transfer procedure, e.g., documentation.

TREATMENT

A patient with a cyst or abscess requires rest and relief from pain with an appropriate analgesia. Antibiotics are often prescribed. Surgical excision of an abscess will provide drainage and relief of symptoms and is performed by a doctor. Swabs should be taken from the abscess for culture and sensitivity and the nurse may be asked to do this. Some abscesses will be due to gonorrhoea.

Unfortunately many abscesses recur. The best treatment for them and for cysts is marsupialization. In *marsupialization* the cyst or abscess is incised and thoroughly drained. The surgical incision is usually made on the inner labial surface. The walls of the cavity are then sutured to the surrounding skin, leaving an open cavity (Fig. 6.2). The cavity may be loosely packed with ribbon gauze impregnated with an antiseptic solution. The normal function of the gland will be retained as a lack of secretion may lead to dyspareunia which is distressing for sexually active women. Occasionally complete excision of a Bartholin's gland may be necessary if cysts or abscesses become chronic.

It is better that a Bartholin's abscess be surgically incised rather than allowing it to burst. If the abscess bursts there may be trauma and it will be more difficult for the function of gland to be retained. The best method to retain the use of the gland is marsupialization. The swelling is usually distorting the posterior labia on the affected side. The pain is such that sitting or walking is agonising. Occasionally pus may be discharging from the swelling. A swab will be taken for

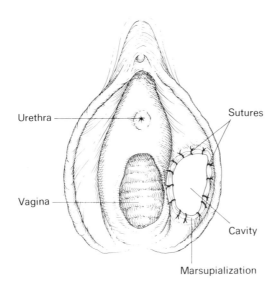

Urethra

Sutures

Vagina

Cavity

Marsupialization

Fig. 6.2. Marsupialization of a Bartholin's abscess.

culture and sensitivity and urine tested for glycosuria. The patient will have been unable to obtain any adequate relief from her pain and may have spent several sleepless nights before seeking medical attention.

NURSING CARE

PREOPERATIVE

The patient needs rest, reassurance and relief from pain; these are priorities. Adequate explanations from the nurse will reduce anxiety; the patient will appreciate knowing that marsupialization is a relatively minor surgical procedure and that hospitalization will be for approximately 48 hours. Analgesics will help the patient to rest once she is free from pain.

To prepare the patient for the operation a vulval shave is excluded because of pain and swelling and the possible distress it may cause the patient. Warm baths, however, will be cleansing and soothing preoperatively. The provision of a sterile vulval pad is necessary if there is a discharge. The nurse must ensure that the patient receives rest prior to theatre.

POSTOPERATIVE

Relief from the severe pain of the abscess is obtained by marsupialization but nevertheless the site will remain tender and painful for several days. Postoperative nursing care will involve a specific plan of care which includes observation of the vulval area and vulval toilet, analgesia and rest for the patient and general management of the wound.

Observation of vulval area

After marsupialization a small ribbon gauge wick impregnated with an antiseptic may be lightly packed into the wound. This should be checked and observed postoperatively.

Vulval toilet

The vulval area must be kept clean—4-hourly vulval toilet is necessary until the patient can bathe. A sterile vulval pad may be applied if the patient finds it comfortable, or if there is a slight oozing from the wound.

Analgesia

Mild analgesia is usually sufficient postoperatively.

Rest

The patient should be allowed to rest in the ward after surgery.

Management of the wound

Any gauge wick is removed after 24 hours—the area remains tender and care should be taken with removal. Often the wick is best 'floated' out whilst the patient is in the bath. Baths twice daily are beneficial.

ON DISCHARGE

The patient is usually allowed home after 48 hours with instructions to maintain vulval hygiene and assist healing by taking frequent baths, at least twice daily. Antibiotics may be prescribed according to the swab culture and sensitivity. There is little chance of a recurrent abscess on the affected side since the cavity has been laid bare.

Infections

Many common pathogens and some parasites may cause a vulval infection and this is especially so if poor standards of hygiene exist, or if the patient is in a state of debilitation. Vaginal infections from trichomonal or monilial organisms are often the cause of vulvitis. Diabetics often experience vulvitis because glycosuria favours the growth of *Candida albicans*.

SYMPTOMS

Pruritus is common, and painful micturition and tender vulva are all experienced as symptoms of vulval infection. Hair follicles may become infected (*folliculitis*) and when the infection becomes more deeply seated the condition is known as *furunculosis*. In furunculosis the base of a hair follicle becomes pus-filled, is extremely painful and difficult to treat.

TREATMENT

Treatment should include tactful education in the principles of good vulval hygiene. Frequent baths should be encouraged and the vulval area gently washed with a weak nonirritating antiseptic soap, or a solution such as hexachlorophane.

Exposure of the vulva to ultraviolet light can be beneficial. The nurse may be asked to take a swab from the vulval region so that an effective antibiotic may be prescribed by the doctor once the culture and antibiotic sensitivity has been established by laboratory methods. This may be necessary if there is a recurrence which often is the case.

Herpes genitalis

Herpes genitalis is vulval infection caused by the herpes II virus, resulting in vesicular eruption with pruritus. The vulva becomes inflamed and extremely tender. Treatment is with an antibiotic dusting powder or the application of gentian violet.

The importance of herpes genitalis is that it may possibly be an aetiological factor in carcinoma of the cervix, as the herpes II virus is believed to irritate the epithelium of the cervix, possibly producing malignant changes. This condition is dealt with in more detail in chapter 2.

Tumours

BENIGN

Benign tumours usually present as a painless lump. This lump may be a:
  Fibromata—arising from fibrous tissue
  Lipoma—a fatty tumour
  Hiradenoma—a rare tumour of the sweat glands
  Sebaceous cyst—arising from a hair
  Condylomata acuminata—vulval warts
  Most of these tumours can be treated by simple excision. Vulval warts (Fig. 6.4) may be treated by an application of podophyllin ointment 25 %. Large warts are best treated by cautery or surgical excision.
NB Podophyllin may cause discomfort and should be removed if this is the case.

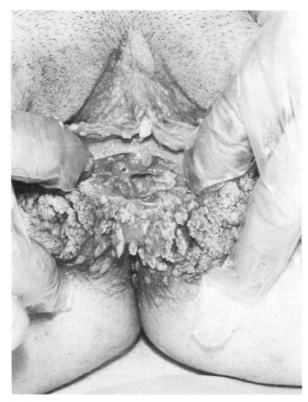

Fig. 6.3. Multiple vulval warts.

MALIGNANT

The importance of full investigation into pruritus vulvae and leucoplakia become even more significant if one considers that a vulval carcinoma **may** be preceded by either condition. Vulval carcinoma is most common in older women, but younger women may be affected.

Nurses have an important role to play in ensuring that any woman complaining of pruritus or other types of vulval irritation seeks the advice of a doctor at the earliest possible moment. I have said earlier that local applications may be tried unsuccessfully for months or even years before a malignant lesion of the vulva is discovered. The most common malignancy of the vulva is a squamous cell carcinoma, which whilst in itself is not common, does account for 95 % of all vulval cancers.

Other malignant tumours include:
    Malignant melanoma
    Rodent ulcer (basal cell carcinoma)
    Adenocarcinoma
    Intraepithelial carcinoma
These are all rare vulval tumours.

Squamous cell carcinoma

The usual site of squamous cell carcinoma (Fig. 6.4) is on the labia majora in the form of an ulcer which may be cauliflower-like in growth or in the form of an excavation. A flattened indurated area may be another presentation of this malignancy.

Diagnosis is based on histological examination. All vulval lumps **must** be biopsied. The age group prone to this malignancy is usually 60-70 years old and the tumour can be symptomless, until it enlarges and begins to bleed or discharge.

SPREAD

There is frequently a direct spread of the carcinoma to the urethra, vagina and anus but far more serious is the spread to the lymphatic glands in the groin. Lymphatic spread results in dissemination of the cancer cells, producing metastases and a poor prognosis. Lymph nodes are involved in up to 50 % of women seen with this condition. The glands involved are the:
    Superficial inguinal
    Deep inguinal (femoral)
    Cloquet's gland in the femoral canal
    Iliac glands
    Aortic glands
This chain of communicating glands form a triangular route.

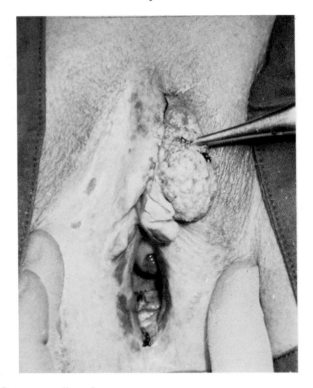

Fig. 6.4. Squamous cell carcinoma.

TREATMENT

The essential treatment is radical vulvectomy (Fig. 6.5) with block dissection of superficial and femoral lymph glands. In the older frail patients this operation will be modified and be more palliative than curative. Radiotherapy may be used for patients unable to withstand surgery, but often cancerocidal dosage causes too many distressing side effects. Shrinkage of the tumour may be achieved with some degree of palliation.

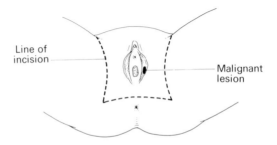

Fig. 6.5. Radical vulvectomy.

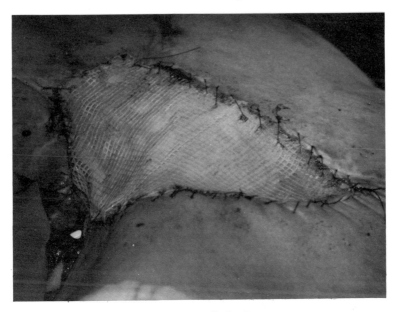

Fig. 6.6.   Excised area skin grafted after a radical vulvectomy.

NURSING CARE

Highly skilled nursing care is required for a patient undergoing a radical vulvectomy. Surgery is prolonged (2-2½ hours) and fluid loss is considerable during
this procedure. Intravenous fluid replacement will be commenced during the
operation and several units of blood may be needed. Shock may be profound and
sepsis is almost inevitable. Hospitalization may be upwards of 12 weeks, and the
psychological trauma of such seemingly mutilating surgery is a considerable factor in the patient's total recovery. More than routine postoperative care is needed.

Environment

A single room is preferable initially because of the intensive nursing care which
is necessary (oxygen and electrical power points must be available). An intravenous infusion stand and a urinary drainage bag stand **must** be available.

Bed

The bed should be adjustable with a ripple or a water-filled mattress, or a
mattress covered in sheep-skin, real or synthetic. A bed-cradle and additional
pillows must be made available.

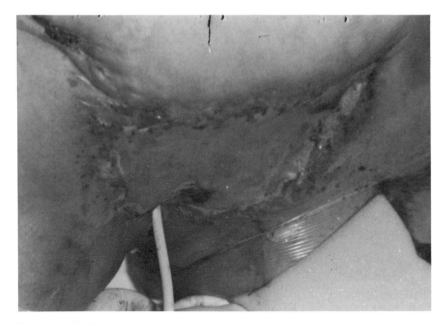

Fig. 6.7.   Healing after skin grafting of a vulvectomy.

Position

On recovery from unconsciousness the patient is probably most comfortable in a recumbent position with two or three pillows. Any strain on the suture line will be painful and must be avoided. Positional change is difficult but modifications of position can be achieved by careful lifting technique and the placement of supporting pillows inbetween the patient's thighs and at her back.

Flowtron boots (calf stimulators) may be in position for several hours following surgery to maintain adequate lower limb circulation.

Bladder drainage

A Foley catheter will be *in situ* and connected to closed continuous drainage. This indwelling catheter may remain in position for up to three weeks. Surgical trauma makes voiding impossible in the early postoperative days and leakage of urine would contaminate the wound. Eventually when healing has taken place spontaneous voiding is possible even though a third to a half of the urethra may have been removed in some cases.

Wound care

The wide excision of tissue necessary in radical vulvectomy means that the wound can only be partially closed leaving a central area open (Fig. 6.6). This granulates and may be skin grafted at a later date (Fig. 6.7). Profuse serous fluid loss from the wound occurs for several days following surgery.

Dressing of the area is difficult and often unsatisfactory. Vacuum drains may be used to collect some of this excessive drainage. A nonadhesive dressing **must** be used such as tulle gras which should be left undisturbed for several days. A gamgee pad secured by a T bandage will provide absorption. These outer dressings must be changed whenever they are saturated.

The most effective way of managing a vulvectomy wound is to allow the patient to take twice daily baths once she is mobilized and granulation of the wound is taking place. Just as sepsis is almost inevitable, sloughing of tissue is also a very common wound problem. If skin grafting is proposed desloughing agents such as Eusol or a solution of Milton will be needed. A heat lamp can be helpful for drying the wound which remains moist because of the continuous serous oozing.

Some surgeons use a surgical technique which allows almost full closure of the wound. The same wide excision of tissue takes place but by using an 'undermining' dissection technique the skin is left intact whilst the underlying tissue is removed (Fig. 6.8). Subcutaneous and deep vacuum drains are inserted at each groin, and vulval drains might be in position. This technique makes the postoperative management much easier, involving much less disturbance for the patient. Serous oozing is greatly reduced, the risk of sepsis is lessened and wound healing a much swifter process. The degree of scar tissue is also reduced and therefore the cosmetic result much more acceptable to the patient.

Mobility

The patient must be mobilized slowly, especially if she is frail or elderly. The aim is to encourage ambulation 72 hours after surgery, but the process must be slow and gradual. Physiotherapy on the other hand must begin immediately after surgery, leg exercises are particularly important, to avoid thrombosis. Oedema of the legs is common following vulvectomy because of interference with lymphatic drainage, but should disappear approximately 12 months after surgery. Postoperatively the patient's legs should be elevated when she sits out of bed.

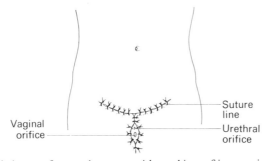

Fig. 6.8. Partial closure after a vulvectomy with no skin grafting required.

Pain relief

Pain and discomfort must be relieved in the usual way by proper use of pain relief drugs so that movement is encouraged. Despite radical surgery the patient experiences much less pain than one would imagine following this procedure.

Psychological effects

Nurses may find that despite the preoperative explanation and psychological preparation given to the patient, the patient may never be completely prepared for what she may regard as the apparently mutilating effects of a radical vulvectomy. She may find it difficult to come to terms with her altered physical appearance. Time must be spent by the nurse in helping her to adjust to her new body image. The psychological effects of radical vulvectomy are comparable to those following mastectomy.

Coital problems

Sexual activity can usually be resumed when complete healing has taken place. Coitus may be difficult because of the loss of labial tissue and stenosis of the vagina from scar formation. Gentleness and understanding from the woman's partner will be necessary during the initial attempts at coitus. In younger women, conception is possible and delivery may take place.

ANATOMY OF THE VAGINA

The vagina is a fibromuscular tube extending from the vestibule to the cervix uteri. The vagina extends upwards and backwards at an angle of approximately 45° to the horizontal and is between 7 cm and 10 cm long, the anterior wall being the shorter (Fig. 6.9). These details need to be considered when taking vaginal specimens. Fixed to this fibromuscular coat is a mucous membrane of stratified epithelium. The epithelium contains glycogen which stains dark brown when iodine is applied. This is a diagnostic sign (see p. 76).

Running longitudinally to the midline of the vaginal walls are two bands of fascia, from these bands, horizontal folds extend laterally—these are called *rugae* (Fig. 6.10). These rugae allow for greater distension of the vagina during childbirth.

The vagina has no secretion of its own as such; there is a fluid transudate from the vaginal mucosa which keeps the vagina moist. Lubrication of the vagina is provided by the Bartholin's glands and glands within the cervix. The pH of the vagina is normally acid. This acidity is of practical importance. The normal pH of the vagina is in the range of 4-5.5. This acid media helps in the resistance of bacterial invasion. A normal inhabitant of the vaginal flora is the Döderlein's

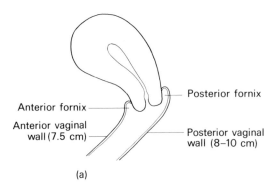

Posterior fornix

Anterior fornix

Anterior vaginal
wall (7.5 cm)

Posterior vaginal
wall (8–10 cm)

(a)

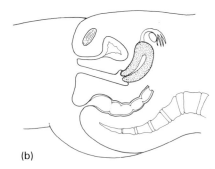

(b)

Fig. 6.9. Length and angle of the vagina (a). The angle when the patient is lying on her back must be considered for internal examination (b).

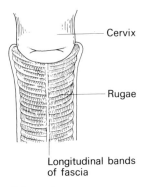

Cervix

Rugae

Longitudinal bands
of fascia

Fig. 6.10. Horiztonal folds of the vagina—rugae.

bacillus which helps to provide acidity of the vagina by converting glycogen to lactic acid.

The vagina at its upper border ends in the vault which is divided into four areas called fornices. The singular being a fornix. These areas are the anterior and posterior fornices and the two lateral fornices (Fig. 6.11). The entrance to the vagina is called the *introitus* and this is covered by the labia. The walls of the vagina are normally in apposition.

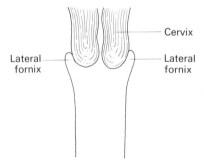

Fig. 6.11   Vaginal fornices.

CONDITIONS OF THE VAGINA

Conditions of the vagina include: senile vaginitis, cysts, carcinoma, fistulae, and imperforate hymen. Vaginal discharge is dealt with in chapter 3.

Senile vaginitis

Atrophic vaginitis is now used in preference to senile vaginitis as it is a more tactful term. The vaginitis is caused by a withdrawal of oestrogen at the time of the menopause. This ultimately lowers glycogen production by the vaginal epithelium and subsequently results in less lactic acid being produced. The pH rises and in this alkaline medium pathogenic invasion becomes more likely.

CLINICAL FEATURES

Discharge may be profuse, offensive and occasionally blood-stained; vulval and vaginal skin may be inflamed. A sample of the vaginal discharge will be taken but no one specific organism isolated.

TREATMENT

Treatment is based on improving the condition of vaginal epithelium and thus restoring vaginal pH to acid. This is done by giving oestrogens either orally (ethinyloestradiol 0.01 mg twice daily) or by local application daily (dienoestrol cream vaginally by applicator). The acidity of the vagina can be improved by inserting a lactic acid pessary vaginally each night. One final point on atrophic vaginitis is that the finding of a blood-stained discharge will demand full investigation to exclude any malignancy of the genital tract.

Cysts

Vaginal cysts are fairly uncommon, they may be congenital and of embryonic origin, or they may be deposits of endometrium which look bluish in colour and which may be painful at the time of menstruation. Vaginal cysts may be symptomless but if the cyst becomes enlarged, it may cause dyspareunia. Treatment is by simple surgical excision or marsupialization.

Carcinoma

Vaginal carcinoma is a rare disease seen mainly in postmenopausal women. Clinical signs include blood-stained vaginal discharge, pain and dysuria.

TREATMENT

Radiotherapy by direct application of radium needles is the treatment of choice. Occasionally if the patient is young extensive surgery may be undertaken. Survival rates, however, are not good.

Fistulae

A *fistula*, which is an abnormal communication between structures, may occur in several places within the genital tract (Fig. 6.12). The opening may be:
    Vesicovaginal
    Urethrovaginal
    Rectovaginal
    Ureterovaginal
    Uterovesical
    Ureteric

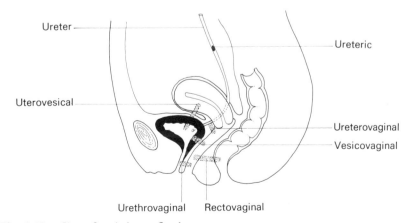

Fig. 6.12. Sites of genital tract fistulae.

The uterovesical and ureteral fistulae do not communicate with the vagina. The most common fistula is vesicovaginal.

The causes of all genital tract fistulae may be summarized as due to obstetric, operative or radiotherapy trauma, or erosion from extensive carcinoma of the cervix. In cases of prolonged or obstructed labour fistula formation is common, this is particularly so in the developing countries. Hysterectomy and vaginal surgery such as anterior colporrhaphy commonly accounts for resultant urethrovaginal and vesicovaginal fistulae. A carcinoma of the cervix may extend both anteriorly or posteriorly to produce vesicovaginal and rectovaginal fistulae. In radiotherapy fistulae formation is usually the result of tissue necrosis.

CLINICAL FEATURES

In nearly all patients with a genital tract fistula the main complaint is that of urinary incontinence. The patient may become very distressed and dejected because she is constantly wet, night and day. In patients with a rectovaginal fistula, faeces may leak into the vagina and in patients with radiotherapy trauma or extensive carcinoma of the cervix both urine and faeces may be leaking into the vagina. This continuous leakage into the vagina and onto the vulva soon produces vaginitis and vulvitis with painful excoriations.

VAGINAL EXAMINATION

The diagnosis may be confirmed by examining the patient vaginally. The patient is helped by the nurse into the Sims's position and a Sims's speculum is inserted into the vagina.

With a urinary tract fistula, urine can be seen to be pouring into the vagina through a small hole in the anterior wall. A rectovaginal fistula can similarly be seen by retracting the anterior vaginal wall so as to visualize the fistula on the posterior wall. Not all fistulae are easily seen. A fistula may be pinpoint in size. A test done to confirm the presence of a small vesicovaginal fistula is the 3 swab test.

Three swab test

The 3 swab test is first explained to the patient. The method involves three cotton wool swabs being inserted into the vagina and the patient catheterized. A nurse may catheterize the patient if asked to do so. The three swabs are carefully positioned; one in the vaginal vault, one midvagina and one at the lower end of the vagina (Fig. 6.13). Methylene blue dye is then instilled into the bladder via the catheter, or given by the intravenous route if a ureteric fistula is suspected.

The results are interpreted thus:

   Lowest swab stains blue = Urethrovaginal fistula
   Middle swab stains blue = Vesicovaginal fistula
   Highest swab is wet = Ureterovaginal fistula

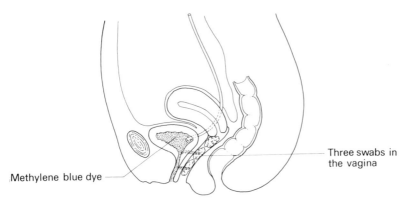

Three swabs in the vagina

Methylene blue dye

Fig. 6.13. The three swab test to demonstrate urethral and vesical fistulae. The upper swab does not become stained with dye.

With a ureterovaginal fistula the swab is stained with urine, as the dye is in the bladder and not the ureter, unless the intravenous instillation is given.

Other diagnostic tests are cystoscopy, intravenous pyelography and retrograde pyelography to locate the site of a urinary fistula.

TREATMENT

Fistulae which have been recently formed during vaginal or abdominal surgery may heal spontaneously. Occasionally this type of fistula may respond to conservative treatment, by passing a Foley catheter and continuously draining the bladder. A low suction pump may facilitate drainage. Bladder drainage will be assisted by nursing the patient in the Sims's or semiprone position. Antibiotics or urinary antiseptics may be prescribed. Care of the vulval area and catheter must be scrupulously attended to. Swabbing the vulva and cleansing the catheter with a weak antiseptic will minimize infection.

Surgical repair is essential as often genitourinary fistulae heal with difficulty. Most fistulae can be repaired through the vaginal wall. A ureterovaginal fistula, however, is usually repaired by the abdominal approach and if much stenosis and fibrosis are found the affected ureter may be reimplanted into the bladder.

NURSING CARE

Nursing care following a fistula repair must include management of fluid intake and urinary output with meticulous attention being paid to catheter care since a self-retaining catheter will remain in position for approximately 12 days. The patient is usually discharged from hospital after 14 days, once spontaneous voiding of urine has been established and residual urine amounts to less than 50 ml.

Imperforate hymen

Any young girl who at puberty complains of lower abdominal pain and is generally not well at monthly intervals, yet has not begun to menstruate, will be examined with the possibility of imperforate hymen in mind. Rarely, when the uterus is distended with old menstrual blood (*haematometra*) a firm swelling can be felt in the pelvis. On external examination, the hymen can be seen bulging at the introitus, it looks bluish in colour. (See Fig. 4.3). This condition has been described briefly in chapter 4.

TREATMENT

Treatment involves excising the hymen with a cross-like incision to allow the escape of old darkened menstrual fluid. Drainage must not be impeded by vaginal packs. Showers rather than baths should be taken so that the risk of an ascending infection is avoided in the following few days. The procedure is done in hospital under a general anaesthetic, and usually the patient remains in hospital until drainage ceases. Vulval hygiene is maintained throughout and often antibiotics are prescribed.

Vaginal examination is best avoided until the young patient is seen as an out-patient. This is because digital examination could cause microorganisms to become present higher up into the reproductive tract, producing infection.

7 The Urethra and Bladder

ANATOMY OF THE URETHRA

The urethra is approximately 4 cm long but may vary from 2 cm to 5 cm. It extends from the external urinary meatus in the vestibule, to the base of the bladder and is about 6 mm in diameter. The urethra follows the line of the vagina and runs upwards and backwards being partially embedded in the anterior vaginal wall. This short, straight tubular structure is made up of involuntary muscle and has a mucous membrane lining. The urethra is moistened by secretion from the paraurethral glands; two tiny structures called Skene's tubules situated at the external meatus of the urethra, drain these glands.

The urethra does not have 'true' anatomical sphincters but the muscle becomes thickened and more complex at certain points. One such point occurs mid-urethra and provides muscular tone and control. This arrangement is called the compressor urethrae or external sphincter.

The urethra is easily distensible which helps during female catheterization. This distensibility may also explain the relative ease with which foreign bodies may be introduced, as occasionally a woman may be seen at the outpatient clinic and be found to have a foreign body lodged in her urethra.

CONDITIONS OF THE URETHRA

The urethra may be subject to various conditions, e.g., urethritis, cystourethritis, caruncles, prolapse, carcinoma, and urethrocele.

Urethritis

Inflammation of the urethra is known as *urethritis* and is caused by an infecting organism. This may be introduced during catheterization of the urinary bladder, a procedure commonly performed in the care of gynaecological patients. Alternatively, the infection may be caused by organisms from adjacent structures which themselves are infected, i.e., Bartholin's abscess, cervicitis or vaginitis. Urethritis may be due to venereal disease with gonococcus found to be the infecting organism (see chap. 11).

Urethritis can be acute or chronic. The Skene's tubules are often sites of chronic urethritis and can be extremely resistant to treatment, and may result in the patient becoming despondent and depressed.

TREATMENT

For acute urethritis, treatment involves the application of:
  Broad spectrum antibiotics.

Treatment for a trichomonal infection—metronidazole (Flagyl).
For chronic urethritis, treatment would involve:
  Urethral instillations of Terra-Cortril (a combination of oxytetracycline and hydrocortisone).
  Dilatation of the stenosis.

Cystitis

When a urethral infection ascends it may cause *cystitis* which is an acute inflammation of the bladder. The symptoms may be acute dysuria and frequency, and are often severe exhausting the patient eventually.

TREATMENT

Treatment for cystitis must include the drinking of copious amounts of fluid (at least 4 litres in 24 hours), pain relief and antibiotics.

Cystourethritis

Infections of the bladder (cystitis) and infections of the urethra (urethritis) may form a complex syndrome known as *urethral syndrome*. This syndrome may include the so called 'honeymoon cystitis' (traumatic urethritis) and urethral and bladder infections caused by a variety of viruses and bacteria, and also by trauma.

The proximity of the urethra to the anus and vagina, and the relatively short length of the urethra probably account for its susceptibility to infection and the nearness of the urethra to the vagina may account for the incidence of trauma at coitus. The incidence of infection and trauma to the bladder and the urethra is intensified when the patient is catheterized especially as this occurs frequently preoperatively and postoperatively. An indwelling catheter increases the risk of infection. Symptoms inlcude frequency, dysuria and possibly some local discomfort or suprapubic pain.

The vulnerability of the urethra is humorously expressed here by F.C. Westerhout Jr MD, an American gynaecologist:

> Oh fair urethra sitting there
> Between the bladder and the air
> Bruised by many an unkind blow
> From fetus passage to libido

TREATMENT

A midstream specimen of urine (MSSU) must be obtained for culture and sensitivity. It is vital to discuss with the patient the origin of her symptoms and whether or not sexual intercourse precedes the onset of symptoms. It may be that coitus causes trauma or introduces infective organisms into the urethra.

PRINCIPLES OF MANAGEMENT

1 High fluid intake.

2 Avoid delaying micturition.

3 Void before and after intercourse—double voiding is effective in preventing residual urine. The woman should void once, then walk around for a little while before voiding again to ensure complete emptying of the bladder.

4 Scrupulous vulval and perineal hygiene.

When symptoms are thought to be caused by the mechanical trauma of coitus, the use of vulval and vaginal lubrication may be beneficial. If these symptoms persist oral preparations, i.e., nitrofurantoin or co-trimoxazole may be prescribed.

Caruncle

A *urethral caruncle* is a small bright red pedunculated 'polyp' found on the posterior margin of the urethral orifice. It is extremely painful to touch and because it is very vascular may bleed. A caruncle may cause dyspareunia and dysuria, and may be painful for the patient when walking or sitting. A urethral caruncle most commonly occurs after the menopause.

TREATMENT

Diathermy to the base of the caruncle is usually sufficient to treat a caruncle. In cases when the caruncle persists, surgical excision of the area may be necessary.

Prolapse

It is the mucous membrane of the urethra which prolapses. The prolapsed mucosa is dark red and because it is vascular, bleeds easily. Urethral prolapse may be confused with a caruncle initially. Unlike a urethral caruncle, however, the prolapsed mucosa is usually seen round the whole circumference of the external meatus.

The symptoms a urethral prolapse causes are similar to those of a caruncle. Dysuria may be severe and there may be complaints of frequency or urgency of micturition. This condition may be seen in childhood or in women who are menopausal.

TREATMENT

Symptoms must be treated and initially an indwelling catheter may be inserted until the tissue oedema subsides. Antiseptic creams may be applied locally and local applications of oestrogenic creams may improve the condition. In the acute stage of urethral prolapse excision of prolapsed mucosa may be necessary.

Carcinoma

Urethral carcinoma is a rare condition, seen mainly in the postmenopausal age group of women. The patient usually complains of dysuria, frequency of micturition and pain. There may be bleeding from the tumour. Unfortunately by the time symptoms present the carcinoma is usually quite well advanced, and the prognosis is poor.

TREATMENT

Implantation of radium needles around the urethral meatus may be successful in the treatment of carcinoma of the external urethra, or wide surgical excision of the vulva and adjacent lymphatic glands may be necessary (see chap. 6). The latter may be employed, but there is no guarantee of a cure. This makes such mutilating surgery hard to justify.

Urethrocele

Since the urethra is embedded in the anterior vaginal wall it follows that if the anterior wall of the vagina is lax and prolapsed that the lower part of the urethra may also prolapse with it. A urethrocele is occasionally associated with a cystocele and uterine prolapse which is described in chapter 8.

The most important and troublesome symptom is a disturbance of micturition, i.e., stress incontinence, and is caused by weakness of the internal sphincter. *Stress incontinence* is the involuntary escape of a small amount of urine when the patient strains or raises her intraabdominal pressure as in coughing or laughing. This kind of incontinence is a great social embarrassment to a woman and as she may be constantly moist in the vulval area there is a risk of a urinary tract infection and local excoriation of vulval tissues. The misery and depressive effect that these symptoms may create should not be underestimated. These psychological disturbances may be profound enough to warrant treatment.

INVESTIGATIONS

Treatment should be preceeded by full urinary tract investigation.
1 Vaginal examination will reveal an anterior wall prolapse.
2 Stress incontinence may be demonstrated during vaginal examination by asking the patient to cough and then witnessing the ejection of a small amount of urine.
3 Cystoscopy and intravenous pyelography will reveal information on function and abnormality.
4 Cystometry will provide a record of dynamic detrusor function.

TREATMENT

Some patients with cystourethrocele may be treated by anterior colporrhaphy which is a repair operation which strengthens and supports the vaginal wall.

This will repair any cystocele which may be present and also restore the anatomy of the urethrovesical junction. Redundant tissue from the lax wall is excised and underlying fascia is tightened by suturing. All of this provides reinforcement for the anterior wall.

Occasionally a simple vaginal repair fails to provide a cure, and other surgical procedures may be used. These will include a vaginal urethroplasty, a fascial sling, a Marshall-Marchetti-Krantz operation or a urethral reconstruction. These are briefly summarized.

A *vaginal urethroplasty* operation is sometimes called 'buttressing' of the urethra, and aims to strengthen and support the urethrovesical angle and urethra. With a *fascial sling* (Aldridge's operation) the principle is to pass a strip of fascia under the urethra at the urethrovesical junction. The fascia is taken from the external oblique muscle. See Garrey *et al.* in suggested further reading for a more detailed coverage of technique. With the *Marshall-Marchetti-Kranz* operation, the principle is to elevate the urethrovesical junction and in some cases the bladder. This is a relatively simple operation approached by suprapubic incision into the space of Retzius just behind the symphysis pubis. The fascia surrounding the urethra and bladder neck is sutured to the back of the symphysis pubis. A *urethral reconstruction* consists of removing old fibrotic or diseased tissue usually from previous surgery, from the urethra and replacing it with a piece of fascia which is usually removed from abdominal muscle.

NURSING CARE STUDY—FASCIAL SLING

Mrs R. is a married lady aged 47 years. She has been admitted to hospital for surgery to correct a long-standing urinary incontinence.

Past history

Mrs R. has suffered urinary incontinence for eight years. Previous vaginal hysterectomy and anterior colporrhaphy in 1980 failed to improve her urinary incontinence. Mrs R.'s obstetric history is Para 3, her three children are all grown up, but still live at home. (Para 3 = three living children).

Urinary symptoms

Mrs R. is incontinent whilst mobile or inactive, she becomes incontinent whilst travelling, sitting or doing her household chores. When her bladder is full she experiences an aching sensation in the perineal region. She does not experience nocturia or dysuria.

On examination she was found to have a lax vaginal introitus, poor pelvic floor contraction and a cystourethrocele. A cystoscopic examination showed a mild trigonitis. A fascial sling operation was scheduled for the next day. The nursing care plan for a patient undergoing this type of operation is shown in Table 7.1.

Table 7.1 Fascial sling—nursing care plan.

Specific problems (potential/actual)	Objectives	Nursing actions
Preoperative Anxiety towards the outcome of surgery.	Establishment of positive attitude towards surgical repair. Reassurance.	Full explanation of post-operative plan. Introduction to other patients recovering successfully from similar surgery. Reinforcement of explanations using simple diagrams if appropriate.
Postoperative Urinary tract infection via Foley catheter (*in situ* for up to 8 days)	Avoid to-and-fro movement of catheter. Prevention of concentrated urine. Maintain urinary acidity. Prevent hospital-acquired infections (nosocomial).	Anchor the catheter to thigh with strapping. Encourage adequate fluid intake 2-3 litres per day. Monitor pH of the urine. Twice daily vulval swabbing and aseptic catheter care (Hexachlorophane)
Urinary retention following removal of indwelling catheter.	Promotion of urinary continence and normal pattern of voiding.	Bladder drill and pelvic floor physiotherapy. Monitor fluid intake and urinary output. Estimation of residual urine.
Vaginal bleeding.	Recognition of excessive blood loss. This will be masked initially as the vaginal pack absorbs the blood until saturated. Avoid straining at defaecation.	Observation of bleeding through any vaginal pack whilst *in situ* and following removal. Regular observations of blood pressure, pulse and respiration. Give faecal softening preparations (e.g., glycerine suppositories).
Wound infection.	Prompt recognition of signs of wound infection necessitating chemo-therapeutic intervention.	Management of wound drains. Monitor amounts and type of drainage. Aseptic technique for wound dressing. Observations (4-hourly) of temperature, pulse and respiration.

Medical assessment

Mrs R. has been seen previously at a 'preoperative' clinic and fully assessed as to her fitness for surgery. Haemoglobin estimation was 12.5 g/dl, 2 units of blood were cross-matched in preparation. Her long history of incontinence and failure of previous surgery to improve matters naturally made her anxious about the outcome of further surgery. An MSSU showed no urinary tract infection at microscopic examination.

Evaluation

The first stage of the surgical procedure was to make an incision into the anterior vaginal wall and free the urethra and bladder neck. The next step was to make an abdominal incision and free two strips of fascia from the external oblique muscle, these strips were then passed under the urethra and sutured together. This then provides a supportive sling for the urethra. The vaginal incision was then closed and a proflavin pack inserted.

Two wound drains were inserted, one in the space of Retzius and one in the subcutaneous tissues. Both were vacuum drains which required regular recharging once vacuum suction was exhausted. Finally the abdominal incision was closed and tension sutures inserted, Michel clips were used as skin closures. Mrs R. returned to the ward with a Foley indwelling catheter *in situ* connected to a closed system continuous drainage. The estimated blood loss during surgery was 500 ml, 2 units of blood previously cross-matched was given.

Following surgery

Special instructions were given to the nursing staff following surgery, on the care of Mrs R. Metronidazole (Flagyl) tablets 200 mg were commenced three times daily, co-trimoxazole (Septrin) tablets 960 mg twice daily and ammonium chloride tablets 1.5 g four times daily. The vaginal pack was to remain *in situ* for 24 hours and the Foley catheter for 8 days. Wound drains were to be removed when drainage was minimal.

Mrs R.'s recovery from her fascial sling operation was satisfactorily progressive. Eight days after surgery when the Foley catheter was removed, Mrs R. was unable to pass urine. This is common following a fascial sling. Despite a programme of bladder drill Mrs R. voided only 10 ml of urine each time and residual urine was 400 ml. Recatheterization and continuous bladder drainage was necessary for a further 48 hours.

Nurse's role

Adequate reassurance is needed during this period as a patient may become demoralized. Following the construction of a urethral sling the patient may be unable to pass urine once the catheter has been removed. This is usually a 'mechanical' fault due to excessive tension of the fascial sling. The difficulty in passing urine may also be due partly to a urinary tract infection. Frequent specimens of urine should be sent to the pathology laboratory for culture, microscopy and sensitivity.

A programme of rehabilitation of the bladder and urethra must be followed by the patient until normal voiding is achieved. Success with bladder drill depends upon regular voiding and careful monitoring of urinary output. The patient is encouraged to void urine 1-2-hourly. Once the stream is started the patient is taught to stop voiding and tense the pelvic floor muscles; the stream can then be continued until voiding is complete. Each amount is carefully measured and charted. The aim of this drill is to improve muscular tone of urethra and bladder.

Small amounts of urine are passed initially (usually 50-200 ml) and estimations of residual urine are necessary, to establish how much urine remains in the bladder immediately after voiding. Catheterization must be done gently with strict attention to asepsis. If large amounts of urine are remaining in the bladder the patient is going into urinary retention and must be recatheterized. Continuous drainage is needed for a further 48 hours, after which time the catheter is removed and the rehabilitation regime restarted. Drugs such as carbachol 2 mg, 4 times a day may be used as mechanical bladder stimulants. Once regular voiding has been established and the residual urine is less than 50-100 ml the patient is ready to return home.

URODYNAMIC INVESTIGATIONS

Women who are suffering from an apparently intractable condition of the urethra or bladder may be seen in a urodynamic unit (UDU) where a very comprehensive examination and investigation of the urinary tract and its function takes place. The objective of these investigations is to detect the cause of any urinary tract abnormality which produces prolonged, frequent and distressing symptoms, e.g., urinary incontinence.

The UDU will aim to develop a thorough, systematic and sympathetic approach to patients who might eventually be diagnosed as having an emotional or psychological problem, which might account for their condition.

Detailed history

A detailed history is taken from each patient and privacy **must** be ensured during the interview. The woman is asked to identify her complaint and describe the nature of it. Weight, menstrual history and details of parity are also carefully noted. Any other relevant abnormalities such as haematuria, cystitis or other urinary symptoms are recorded. Details of previous vaginal operations, i.e., colporrhaphy and bladder neck surgery, complete the interview.

Techniques of interviewing are particularly important, for whilst very detailed questioning of the patient is necessary, it must be done in a sensitive fashion. Much of the questioning time will be spent discovering the woman's urinary habits. Some of this essential information may be obtained by giving the patient a booklet which she might complete at home. She will be asked to record the time of each visit to the lavatory, night and day; the amount of urine passed each time and whether she was incontinent prior to voiding. This information is gathered over a period of several weeks.

Medical examination

Once the basis for examination and investigation has been established, a medical examination is undertaken and conditions which may contribute to urinary incontinence, i.e., obesity and chronic cough, are noted.

Vaginal examination will reveal the presence of a cystocele, urethrocele, enterocele, rectocele or uterine descent and conditions such as atrophic vaginitis and vulvitis will be seen.

The strength of pelvic floor muscles can be determined by asking the patient to tense her buttocks so that muscle contraction can be felt. Stress incontinence may be demonstrated at this stage of the examination (see p. 89).

Further investigations

A midstream specimen of urine (MSSU) and a catheter specimen of urine (CSU) will be obtained for culture and microscopy so that any urinary tract infection may be excluded or detected. *Cystometry*, measurements of bladder capacity (normal 500-700 ml), filling pressure and residual urine are then recorded and by these means detrusor (bladder muscle) instability can be assessed. Any other cystometric findings, i.e., voiding pressure, are also noted. Sphincter pressures are monitored (*sphincterometry*) and the functional length of the urethra estimated (*urethrometry*). Finally *cystoscopy, urethroscopy* and possibly intravenous *pyelography* complete the investigations.

Diagnosis

Sufficient information may now be at hand to allow a diagnosis to be made. The condition may be due to:

A bladder fault
A sphincter fault
An infection
Urethral stenosis
Fistulae
Cystocele
Urethrocele
Emotional/psychiatric causes
Other causes still be be determined

Patient counselling

The patient will be psychologically prepared for all investigations and time will be spent afterwards advising the patient on how her urinary symptoms may be improved or cured. Both the doctor and the nurse will be involved in this, with the nurse reinforcing the advice given. Treatment will be symptomatic and some of the specific regimens are mentioned later in this chapter.

A follow-up will be arranged and the patient encouraged to contact the department whenever she feels she would like to discuss her progress.

URODYNAMIC STUDIES

Urodynamic studies must now be considered an important and developing subspecialty of gynaecology. It provides a scientific basis for the diagnosis and treatment of urinary tract abnormalities.

Few urodynamic units exist in the United Kingdom but those which function within a teaching hospital, such as at St. Mary's in Manchester, are developing their criteria for treating various conditions diagnosed by urodynamic studies. Research is continuous and because this subspecialty to gynaecology is developing it is appropriate to mention some of the more specific programmes of treatment, developed at St Mary's UDU.

Atrophic urethritis

CLINICAL FEATURES

The first onset of persistent symptoms of atrophic urethritis occur postmenopausally, presenting for longer than 6 months. Some of these are mentioned earlier in this chapter, but in addition hot flushes, vulval soreness and suprapubic pain may exist.

The signs may include:
 Tender urethra
 Atrophic vagina/vulva
 Urethral thickening
 Prolapse
 Vaginal scarring/urethral narrowing

TREATMENT

Treatment will involve precise instructions to the patient regarding vulval hygiene. A dienoestrol cream will be prescribed, to be used vaginally each night for 2 months. Dilatation of the urethral stenosis will take place at 2-monthly intervals, usually on a gynaecological ward, under a general anaesthetic.

If there is no response to this schedule of therapy oral hormone replacement therapy (HRT) may be started. If the urethritis remains unresponsive double-strength co-trimoxazole (Septrin, low dosage long-term for 3-6 months) may be prescribed or a urinary antimicrobial agent such as hexamine (Mandelamine).

If this treatment fails to achieve a cure, reinvestigation will commence.

Stress incontinence

Uncomplicated stress incontinence occurs with raised intraabdominal pressure. The onset is simultaneous with the pressure increase, and ceases when the pressure drops. This incontinence must be demonstrable on examination, and the following conditions noted:

    Cystocele/cystourethrocele
    Uterine/vault prolapse
    Urethral rigidity
    Vaginal capacity and condition
    Pelvic floor muscle tone
Obesity, chronic cough and smoking-habits of the patient will also be recorded.

TREATMENT

In the absence of a prolapse a nonsurgical approach is tried. This includes a reducing diet if obesity exists, hormone replacement therapy in postmenopausal women and physiotherapy in younger women. Follow-up continues for at least 1 year.

If the woman fails to respond to the measures outlined or has symptoms which are associated with prolapse, one of the following surgical repairs will be indicated:

    Urethroplasty with or without anterior colporrhaphy
    Marshall-Marchetti-Krantz operation
    Fascial sling procedures
    Martius graft and fascial patch (in refractory cases)

Mixed incontinence

Mixed incontinence is urinary incontinence due to detrusor instability and sphincter weakness.

SYMPTOMS

The history of mixed incontinence can be confusing as it may have more than one cause. Symptoms may include:

    Provoked or unprovoked incontinence with urgency
    Enuresis
    Frequency/hesitancy
    Dysuria/suprapubic pain
Provoked incontinence occurs on physical effort, e.g., coughing, whilst unprovoked occurs due to anatomical malformation. On examination the patient will

be found to have easily demonstrable stress incontinence and abnormal detrusor function. Neurological examination is necessary to exclude neuropathology, as well as all the previously mentioned urodynamic investigations.

Treatment ranges from conservative, i.e., a weight-reducing diet, physiotherapy (pelvic floor exercises), hormone therapy, to surgical repair of the sphincter weakness. In the case of a neurological disorder, urinary diversion may be considered, if treatment for the disorder is not possible.

There is an increasing awareness that the incontinent patient needs more sympathetic and caring support. To meet this need many new groups and incontinence societies have been established. Facilities have been made in most areas for patients to obtain incontinence pads, pants and other items of protective clothing.

Bladder training

The aim of bladder training is to inhibit micturition. This programme suggested by the UDU at St Mary's hospital, Manchester has a well defined criteria for patient selection. There must be: an inability to inhibit causing incontinence, an absence of a central nervous system disease, an absence of inflammatory lesions of bladder and urethra, and no obstruction to flow.

Treatment

Two approaches are used for treatment: supportive and authoritative. On an outpatient basis, *supportive* treatment involves retraining by the use of psychotherapy and micturition charts. When *authoritative* treatment is applied the patient is admitted to hospital so that urinary control is enforced by the clock. The success rate is approximately 80 % with both methods, at present.

Method

The success of both supportive and authoritative bladder training depends upon indepth discussion with the patient regarding the nature of the problem. Time must be spent in reassuring the patient that no serious organic disease exists and that surgical treatment is not contemplated. If the patient is tense, anxious or emotionally unstable, appropriate drug therapy will be prescribed.

The patient is instructed how to measure and record her urinary output. The patient needs positive reinforcement throughout training and this is achieved by using a drug called phenazopyridine hydrochloride (Pyridium) which colours the urine orange. Evidence of progress is seen by the patient as less and less Pyridium-stained urine appears on her pad. She will then keep a chart of her progress and be encouraged as the amounts decrease. Initially the patient is given the following authoritative instructions:

1 Do not void more frequently than 1½-hourly (the patient is to wait or be incontinent).

2 Initially ignore any nocturnal frequency.

3 When the 1½-hour target has been achieved increase the interval by half-an-hour until voiding takes place 4-hourly.

When this 4-hour target has been reached cystometry is repeated and the patient discharged. The follow-up and continued encouragement are essential. The patient is first seen on a weekly basis for 2 weeks, then at monthly intervals. Bladder charts are kept by the patient for 24-hours prior to appointments. After a follow-up lasting 6 months the patient may be discharged if she is cured.

Summary

Many other conditions are investigated and treated at the UDU such as neuropathic bladder, chronic cystitis, chronic urethritis and underactive detrusor function. The format of therapy remains the same with a thorough systematic investigation, treatment of causative factors and symptomatic treatment. Success also depends on patience, persistence and a sympathetic yet positive approach to the patient. Once the patient is given an insight into her problem she is more likely to appreciate the rationale behind treatment and cooperate willingly and cheerfully.

8 The Uterus

ANATOMY

The uterus is a hollow, thick-walled muscular organ, shaped like a pear and approximately the size of a pear. The measurements of the uterus are clinically important as an increase in the size may indicate some abnormality. These measurements are approximately:

Length	7.5 cm
Breadth (at the superior part)	5.0 cm
Thickness	2.5 cm

The uterus lies in the pelvis inbetween the bladder and the rectum. It tilts forward over the bladder and is said to be anteverted. This position of anteversion is maintained by the round ligaments which arise from in front of and below the uterine tubes and pass through the inguinal canal to the labia majora. The uterus is made up a neck (cervix), a body (corpus), and a fundus (Fig. 8.1).

The cervix

The *cervix* is composed of muscle and fibrous tissue. It communicates with the vagina, via the *external os*, a small rounded opening of the cervix which alters shape after childbirth (Fig. 8.2). The external os communicates with the internal os via the cervical canal, which in turn opens into the uterine cavity. This cervical canal is lined with columnar epithelium and is referred to as the endocervix. The epithelium forms cervical glands which secrete mucus, part of normal vaginal discharge. The surface of the cervix is covered with stratified squamous epithelium. The cervix projects a little way into the vagina, this is known as the *portio vaginalis* or vaginal portion of the cervix.

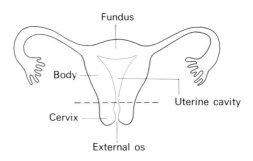

Fig. 8.1. Divisons of the uterus.

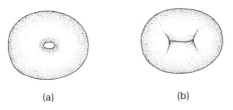

Fig. 8.2. The opening of the cervix, the os: nulliparous os (a), parous os (b).

The corpus

The *corpus* (Fig. 8.3) is made up of thick muscular walls called *myometrium* which form a triangular cavity, the uterine cavity. This *uterine cavity* is lined by a glandular mucous membrane called *endometrium* which is shed monthly at menstruation. The uterus itself is covered by peritoneum which is closely adherent (*perimetrium*) The myometrium is made up of muscle fibres which run in circular, longitudinal and criss-cross fashion. This arrangement enables powerful contractions to be set up at childbirth and also assists in haemostasis.

The fundus

The fundus (see Fig. 8.1) is the upper rounded portion of the uterus which lies above the uterine tubes which communicate directly with the uterine cavity. In pregnancy the fundus can be palpated to estimate the size of the uterus as the fetus grows.

Uterine supports

The uterus is well-supported and positioned by several ligaments which are either fibrous bands of tissue or folds of peritoneum. They are the ligaments of

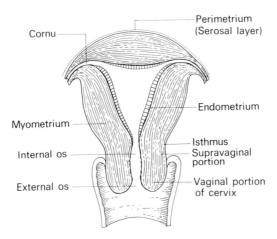

Fig. 8.3. Coronal uterine section.

the pelvis. The *round ligament* maintains anteversion of the uterus. The *broad ligament* is a fold of peritoneum draped over the uterus anteriorly and posteriorly, enclosing the uterine tubes. This ligament has a steadying effect on the uterus. The *cardinal* or *Mackenrodt's ligament* prevents descent of the uterus, by fanning out from the cervix to the pelvic side walls. The *uterosacral ligament* is a posterior extension of this and the *pubocervical ligament* an anterior extension which also prevents descent.

The muscles of the pelvic floor also provide support for the uterus and these as well as the exact arrangement of the supporting ligaments are shown on p. 121. Much of gynaecological surgery is concerned with these structures and their precise function should be understood.

The blood supply to the uterus is via the uterine artery which takes a coiled and tortuous path within the uterine muscle (Fig. 8.4). This is to allow for extension in its length as the uterus grows in pregnancy. The uterine artery continues to anastomose with the ovarian artery and also supply the uterine tube.

CARCINOMA OF THE CERVIX

After breast cancer, carcinoma of the cervix is the second most common malignant disease in women. It occurs more commonly in women of the 40 to 55 age group but increasingly the age scale is shifting to include much younger women.

Cervical carcinoma is largely a preventable disease but if undetected has a 50 % mortality rate. Factors which appear to influence the development of cervical carcinoma are related to sexual intercourse at an early age; virgins rarely develop cancer of the cervix, whilst girls having their first babies when very young are in the 'at risk' group. Promiscuity of both partners increases the risk of cervical cancer.

Several theories implicate smegma as being possibly carcinogenic to the cervix and circumcision is mooted as a practice which may prevent cervical cancer. Jewish women who are orthodox and observe the law of Niddah which does not allow intercourse during menstruation, for 7 days after menstruation or during pregnancy when the cervical epithelium is most at risk, and the postpartum period, seem relatively immune to cancer of the cervix.

Socioeconomic status is another factor to consider as the incidence of cervical

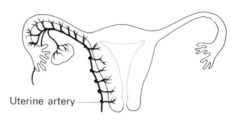

Uterine artery

Fig. 8.4.   Blood supply to the uterus, uterine tubes and ovaries.

cancer increases in lower social groups. Poor standards of hygiene and housing may also contribute to the prevalence of this disease.

Another suspected carcinogen is the herpes virus II (genitalis) which may be capable of penetrating the cervical epithelium and producing local irritation possibly predisposing to malignant changes in the cervical tissue. Whatever the cause of carcinoma of the cervix it *can* be diagnosed whilst still in the premalignant stage, and because of this has a *potentially* high cure rate.

Stages

Cervical carcinoma can be clinically classified into five different stages. Stages I to IV are depicted in Fig. 8.5.

Stage O: Carcinoma *in situ* or, more recently, cervical intraepithelial neoplasia (CIN) a term more descriptive of pathological changes. The histological descriptions of this stage include terms such as:
   Metaplasia—normal transformation of cellular tissue
   Dysplasia—abnormal development or growth of cells: mild (CIN 1), moderate (CIN 2), or severe (CIN 3)
   Dyskaryosis—abnormality of the nuclei of cells.
These terms denote cellular changes which can be seen in the cervical epithelium, but there is no invasion to the deeper tissues. These conditions do not *invariably* progress to a malignancy.

Stage I: The lesion is invasive but confined to the cervix usually at the squamo-columnar junction.

Stage II: The lesion extends beyond the cervix to the upper vagina and parametrium, but not to the pelvic side walls.

Stage III: The lesion reaches one or both pelvic side walls and the lower third of the vagina, whether as a continuous or separate process.

Stage IV: In this stage the spread involves the bladder and/or the rectum. There may also be distant metastases.

Obviously the prognosis becomes worse as the stage of the disease progresses. So that stages 0-I offer a good prognosis whilst in stages III-IV the prognosis is poor despite radical treatment.

Diagnosis

CERVICAL CYTOLOGY (AYRE'S SMEAR)

Cervical cytology is an examination of the cervical cells which are exfoliated constantly into the vagina. These cells are degenerating and are shed from the

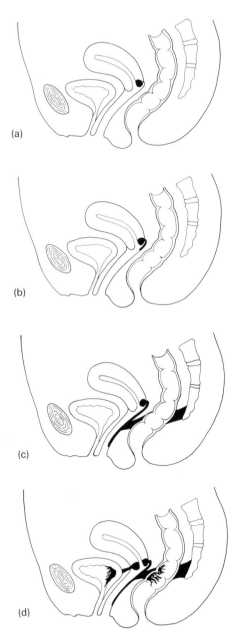

(a)

(b)

(c)

(d)

Fig. 8.5. Stage of cervical carcinoma: stage I is confined to the cervix (a); stage II involves the cervix and the upper vagina (b); stage III involves the cervix and upper and lower third of the vagina, the parametrium and the pelvic side walls (c); stage IV, as in stage III including the bladder and the rectum (d).

epithelium of the cervix. The exfoliated cell may be collected by a wooden Ayre's spatula which is specially shaped to fit into the external os (chap. 2). Lubricants must *not* be used.

The cost of cervical cytology is relatively low compared to other diagnostic tests and it seems that since preinvasive lesions can be discovered by this means it should be done whenever a woman presents herself for gynaecological examination (within a time span of 2-3 years). All postnatal patients should have cervical screening as a routine measure, if not already done in the antenatal period. The age group of women who should have regular cervical cytology is thought to range from mid-twenty to early sixty but there is evidence to support the need to do cytology on much younger women. This relates to the early age of sexual activity.

VAGINAL CYTOLOGY

The method of vaginal cytology has already been mentioned as the vaginal aspiration technique or Papanicolaou's test (see chap. 2). It is a technique that is more likely to detect endometrial cells than cells from the cervix so that as an aid to diagnosis of cancer of the cervix is less efficient than cervical cytology.

COLPOSCOPY

The colposcope, which was invented by a German gynaecologist, has been used in gynaecology since the 1920s. In 1927 Schiller introduced his iodine staining technique. Since then colposcopic work has developed and become highly specialized. Essentially the colposcope is a binocular microscope with a powerful light source and offers a magnification of ×6 to ×40. Today it is a sophisticated piece of equipment incorporating light filters, and photographic attachments. More recently the colposcope has been designed to incorporate the use of laser therapy. With colpomicroscopy magnification of × 100 to × 300 can be achieved.

Nurses have an essential role to play in a colposcopy clinic and an understanding of the sequence of events during colposcopic examination will help to ensure that adequate preparation and support of the patient takes place. The examination may seem to be a lengthy procedure to the patient and she may be anxious if she is not reassured throughout. Effective support can best be given if the nurse stands at the head of the examination couch once positioning and draping of the patient has taken place. From this position she can observe the patient's reactions throughout.

Equipment

On the top shelf of the trolley the following equipment should be prepared:
    Gallipots and lotions
        Normal saline
        Acetic acid 2 % W/V
        Schiller's iodine

Cusco's speculae
Cottonwool swabs
Sponge forceps
Cervical cytology set (wooden and plastic spatulae)
High vaginal swabs
On the bottom shelf, the following should be available:
Receivers
Punch biopsy forceps
Sterile vulval pads
Receptacles for biopsy specimens
Histology and cytology forms

Procedure

Colposcopy and punch biopsy are procedures which can be performed in the outpatient department with little risk of complications developing. A gynaecological history is taken prior to the examination. The patient is then positioned on an examination couch with her feet in the stirrups and her buttocks well towards the edge. Adequate draping of the vulva and perineum will help to make the patient feel less exposed. The colposcope is conveniently placed so that it can be manoevered into position and it's light switches easily manipulated by the operator.

A Cusco's speculum is inserted into the vagina so that naked eye inspection of the cervix can be made; obvious lesions such as an *ectopy* (endocervical mucosa outside its normal boundaries) can be seen. A repeat smear and high vaginal swab may be taken at this point.

The cervix is viewed through the colposcope which provides a concentrated beam of light and magnification of ×6 to ×40. The usual magnifications are ×6, ×10 and ×16. A solution of normal saline is used to swab the cervix so that excessive mucous is cleared. Vascular patterns and any vascular transformation zones may be clearly visible.

The next stages of colposcopic examination are:
1 Acetic acid 2 % W/V is applied to the cervix; this gives greater definition to the area. Abnormal and immature metaplastic epithelium becomes white (acetowhite) at this stage.
2 Schiller's test is then performed. The cervix is again swabbed, this time with Schiller's iodine (this may sting slightly so the patient must be prepared). Any sensitivity to iodine must be excluded. The result is that normal cervical epithelium contains glycogen which will take up the brown stain while the abnormal or malignant tissue contains no glycogen and therefore fails to stain. The stained area will be assessed and from any well-defined area which fails to stain small biopsies can be taken so that histological examination can be carried out.

A decision can eventually be made regarding treatment or further investigation. It may be that a lesion can be treated by laser surgery or cone biopsy or that no treatment other than continued observation is necessary.

To end the procedure the patient is provided with a vulval pad and helped down from the examination couch. She is then allowed to dress before her questions are answered and any proposed treatment is explained carefully to her. It is vital for the patient to understand the situation, she must not be allowed to leave the clinic in a worried state of mind. She should be prepared to expect a slight amount of vaginal bleeding if biopsies have been taken.

CONE BIOPSY

Cone biopsy is a surgical procedure which requires admission to hospital. It involves excision of a cone-shaped piece of cervical tissue. In nulliparous women or women who desire more children a shallow cone avoiding the internal os is taken; in women whose family is complete a more tapered cone which reaches the internal os is removed (Fig. 8.6). In both cases the squamocolumnar junction and a portion of the cervical canal is removed.

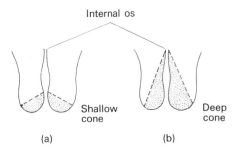

Fig. 8.6. Cone biopsy: from a nulliparous cervix (a), from a multiparous cervix (b).

A cone biopsy will provide histological diagnosis and *may* also remove the whole of the abnormal cervical tissue. A cone biopsy therefore may be both diagnostic and curative. This operation is a relatively simple procedure but it may result in several complications such as cervical stenosis or cervical incompetence, infection may lead to secondary haemorrhage. I have nursed several patients who have haemorrhaged profusely in the immediate postoperative period.

It is essential to maintain postoperative observations of pulse rate and blood pressure hourly for the first 6 hours. The vulval area and pad should be inspected frequently for signs of vaginal bleeding. A vaginal pack may have been inserted in theatre and this is usually removed after 24 hours. It is wise to confine the patient to bed for 24-48 hours.

FURTHER INVESTIGATIONS

Other investigations which may detect metastatic spread include:
    Chest X-ray
    Full blood count and haemoglobin

Cystoscopy

Blood urea

Intravenous pyelography

CAT scan (computerized axial tomography) and lymphangiography

It is vital to know the degree of urinary tract involvement and spread to other tissues before a programme of treatment is planned.

Clinical features

In the early stages of the disease there may be no signs or symptoms and the condition may simply be discovered by routine cervical cytology, even then the cervix may look normal to the naked eye.

Contact bleeding is one of the earliest and most important signs. It may occur after intercourse (postcoital bleeding), after examination or it may occur after the menopause (postmenopausal bleeding). Bleeding may seem to be related to periods or the 'change of life' and unfortunately this may lead to considerable delay before medical advice is sought.

Other features may include vaginal discharge, this may be profuse and offensive, and pain. Pain is a late feature and is indicative of spread beyond the cervix itself. It is usually severe and radiates down the legs. Weight loss, loss of appetite, faecal and urinary incontinence may be experienced if the bladder and rectum are invaded. Finally lymphatic oedema may result from lymphatic obstruction. When the patient is examined the cervix may bleed and the word *friable* is used to describe the texture of the cervix. The cause of death in women who are suffering from a cervical cancer, which has invaded pelvic structures, is usually renal failure and ureamia.

Great nursing skill is required to ensure that the patient is made comfortable. This patient will be emaciated and cachectic. Priorities will include vulval hygiene and management of pain relief. Every effort must be made to restore the patient's morale, possibly offering spiritual support if acceptable or requested by the patient. Nursing staff must also care for the patient's relatives who will be extremely distressed watching their loved one's gradual deterioration. Relatives should be encouraged to participate in the care of this patient.

Treatment

The best results from treatment will be achieved by consultation between a gynaecologist and radiotherapist and often a combination of surgery and radiotherapy may be appropriate.

CARCINOMA *IN SITU*

A carcinoma *in situ* (CIN 3) may be treated by a cone biopsy but often in women who have completed their family a total hysterectomy with removal of the cuff of the vagina may be performed after the diagnosis has been established. The ovaries may be conserved.

INVASIVE CARCINOMA

The treatment of invasive carcinoma depends on the extent of the disease and the age and general condition of the patient.

Radiotherapy

Radiotherapy may be used for all stages of the disease although palliative in stage IV.

Surgery

Surgery may be selected in women with early stages of the disease, who are thought to be able to withstand radical surgery. Wertheim's hysterectomy and lymphadenectomy involves removal of the uterus, both tubes and ovaries, upper third to a half of the vagina, pelvic cellular tissue and regional lymph nodes. The ovaries may be conserved in a young woman.

Pelvic exenteration is radical surgery but offers the only real hope of cure for these women. The operation involves removal of the uterus, tubes, ovaries, pelvic cellular tissue, the vagina and bladder or rectum (or both depending on spread). This means that the ureters have to be transplanted into an ileal loop and if the rectum is removed a colostomy fashioned.

Whatever the final choice of treatment the patient and her partner must be fully involved in the discussion and able to understand what each option entails. In radical surgery she should be aware that if the vagina is removed her sexual activity will be affected. This is an important point for both the woman and her partner to appreciate before consent is obtained.

Application of radiotherapy

Radiotherapy for carcinoma of the cervix may be by direct application of radium or other radioactive source, or by external radiation of the pelvis by super voltage X-rays. Direct radium will be cancerocidal to the tumour whilst X-ray therapy will destroy cancer cells which may have affected pelvic lymph glands.

DIRECT APPLICATION

Methods of application of radioactive substances are based on the principle of insertion into the uterine cavity and the vaginal fornices. The Stockholm and Manchester techniques are commonly employed. Radium, cobalt or caesium are the substances used. The dosage is precisely calculated and varies according to the size and spread of the tumour. Whichever substance is used, and in Manchester it is usually radium, it is enclosed in rubber or perspex.

The uterine applicator is inserted through the cervical canal into the uterine cavity and the ovoids are positioned in the lateral fornices, separated by the spacer (Fig. 8.7). A vaginal pack is inserted to secure the applicators and occasionally the labia are sutured together to afford extra, temporary security. The applicators stay in position until the tumour is destroyed by radiation, usually up to 6 days. Careful checks are made, by inserting a probe attached to a dose meter into the urethra and rectum, to ensure that these structures are not subjected to overdosage. Finally the pelvis is X-rayed to establish correct positioning of the radium applicators.

NURSING CARE

The patient is admitted to hospital as an inpatient 24-48 hours prior to radium treatment, if possible. This gives time for the patient to be prepared and become familiar with her environment. Constant reassurance is essential to help dissipate anxiety. A positive attitude regarding the efficiency of receiving radium by insertion will be encouraging for the patient, and an explanation of the sequence of events will allow the patient to prepare psychologically for her therapy.

Plan of preparation

The patient ideally should be nursed in a single room, or in an end bed placed near a wall (some distance from premenopausal women if possible). The black and yellow symbol denoting radiation should be placed on the bed or the door.

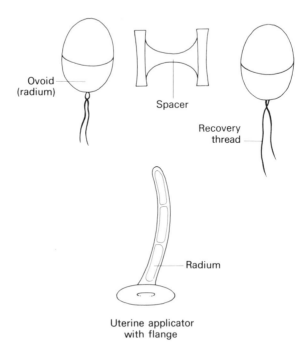

Fig. 8.7. Radium applicators.

The patient will have her pubis, vulva and perineum shaved and then asked to bathe. A preparation will be given to empty the bowel so that defaecation is prevented after insertion of radium. A good night's rest should be obtained. A night sedation may be prescribed to ensure this, particularly if the patient is anxious. The usual preoperative fasting regimen is observed.

Postinsertion

Adequate explanation of the postinsertion management will both reassure the patient and enlist her cooperation.

Specific nursing care

1 Safety precautions must include having long-handled forceps and a lead-lined box available, should the applicators fall out.
2 When the patient returns from theatre she should be carefully positioned on her back with one or two pillows.
3 The patient must be asked to avoid excessive movement so as to prevent dislocating the applicators.
4 Essential exercises which must be encouraged are deep breathing and leg movements. These should be supervized.
5 The patient will have an indwelling catheter *in situ* on continuous drainage.

Nursing observations

1 Temperature, pulse and respiration should be recorded 2-hourly. A pyrexia may indicate an adverse reaction to the radium.
2 Regular checks on vaginal bleeding and the position of the applicators.
3 Urinary output via the catheter must be monitored. Oliguria may be a complication.
4 Nausea and vomiting if observed must be reported. Antiemetics will be prescribed to prevent retching.
5 Pain—should not be severe and must be reported if it is so. Mild analgesia is usually sufficient to ease any discomfort.

Daily nursing care

1 Washing or bedbathing will refresh the patient, and encourage physiotherapy.
2 Swabbing of vulval and perineal areas will remove any unpleasant vaginal discharge. A perineal pad should be worn.
3 Catheter care must include cleansing of the catheter to help prevent a urinary tract infection.
4 Pressure area care is essential whilst the patient is nursed at bedrest. Again excessive or energetic movement must be avoided.

General care

Proper management of the patient's bowel function is an important part of care.
A low residue diet will confine the bowels and avoid straining or defaecation,
which may dislodge the applicators. Occasionally however diarrhoea may be a
complication and an antidiarrhoea preparation such as kaolin may be prescribed.

All nursing care is carried out as quickly as possible so that nurse/patient contact is minimal. Visitors are asked to visit for short periods and keep a distance of
6 feet from their relative. Pregnant women of course should not visit because of
the risk to the fetus. All this will seem to isolate the patient at a time when she
needs extra sympathy and support so advantage must be taken during nursing
procedures to comfort the patient and give moral support.

REMOVAL OF APPLICATORS

Radium applicators are left in position for periods of up to 72 hours. In some
centres the total dose time is divided with weekly intervals between insertions.
Instructions for the time of removal will be precise and recording of removal
must be equally precise. Two nurses must be involved and the time of removal
noted in the case notes followed by a signature. The nursing Kardex must contain this information also.

Technique for removal

A premedication may be prescribed and it should be given in time for it to be effective prior to removal of the radium. The patient must be given a full
explanation of the procedures involved. It will be necessary to assemble equipment for:

Removal of any sutures
Removal of vaginal pack
Vulval and perineal swabbing

The patient is placed in a comfortable position—on her back with her knees
flexed, heels together and thighs abducted. If the labia are sutured together the
sutures are removed. The vaginal pack is removed and then using long-handled
forceps the recovery threads of the ovoids and uterine applicator are grasped and
removed in turn by gentle traction. Both ovoids and uterine applicators are
placed immediately in the lead box, and returned to the radium curator who will
account for the exact amounts.

The indwelling catheter may now be removed and the vulva and perineum
swabbed; a clean perineal pad is applied. The patient is then left resting comfortably. Continued observation of the patient is necessary because there is a risk of
bleeding following removal of the radium applicators.

EXTERNAL APPLICATION

If a patient is receiving external radiation through X-ray therapy to the pelvis
either in addition to intracavity radium or as the means of treating more advan-

ced cases it is vital to realize that the skin shows a very early reaction to excess irradiation. This is especially so in the tissues around the groin and vulva. The effects of irradiation are quite obvious, progressing through:

Redness (erythema)

Scaliness (dry desquamation)

Loss of skin (wet desquamation)

Tissue death (necrosis)

Necrosis is a very extreme tissue reaction which is usually avoided.

NURSING CARE

During treatment the skin must be kept dry if possible. A light dusting powder may be used to keep the patient comfortable but the powder should not contain zinc as powders containing metals affect X-ray treatment. If the patient does need bathing the area receiving treatment must be thoroughly dried. If any skin reaction is obvious the application of Betnovate cream or a solution of gentian violet will help to relieve discomfort.

X-ray therapy may cause distressing symptoms due to bladder irritation. It is important to observe the patient for signs of nocturia, dysuria and urgency.

OTHER CONDITIONS OF THE CERVIX

Cervical erosion and cervicitis, cervical ectropion and polypi are other conditions of the cervix.

Cervical erosion

Cervical erosion is a misnomer as an erosion is not an ulcer, but a red velvety area appearing at the external os. It is an outgrowth of columnar epithelium from the endocervix (or cervical canal) and not an ulceration. An erosion often occurs after *chronic cervicitis* but is common in women who take the contraceptive pill and in pregnant women; it is associated with oestrogenic effects.

CLINICAL FEATURES

Many erosions are symptomless but a serous or mucoid discharge may be experienced. Postcoital bleeding may be experienced and occasionally bleeding occurs after scraping the cervix for cervical cytology. In chronic cervicitis inflammatory changes can be seen. Many Nabothian follicles appear, these are cervical glands which have become distended and are of bluish appearance. Low backache and dyspareunia may be caused by chronic cervicitis.

Ectropion

If the cervix is traumatized during delivery *ectropion*, a laceration of the anterior and posterior lips of the cervix, may occur. Eversion of these lacerations exposes the endocervical canal, which may cause vaginal discharge and slight bleeding.

TREATMENT

A cervical smear must be done in all cases to exclude a cervical carcinoma. Erosions, chronic cervicitis and ectropion can all be treated by either diathermic cauterization or by cryosurgery. *Cryosurgery* involves the application of carbon dioxide, under pressure, to the affected area; this freezes and destroys the tissue. After treatment the cervix soon regenerates. These conditions can also be treated by conization, in which a cone shaped piece of tissue can be removed with a triangular or ring-shaped electrode. These treatments are best done under general anaesthesia.

When the patient is allowed home she should be advised that vaginal bleeding may occur when the diathermized tissue sloughs off. For this reason coitus and the use of vaginal tampons is best avoided for up to 10 days. If vaginal bleeding occurs and is heavy she must be advised to contact her GP or hospital.

Polyps

Polyp formation may occur in association with chronic cervicitis and erosions. They arise from the mucous membrane lining of the cervical canal, hence the name mucous polyp. Vaginal bleeding is a common symptom especially after coitus.

TREATMENT

Treatment consists of twisting the polyp on its stalk until it is avulsed (torn away). Since on rare occasions the polyp might have undergone malignant change it must be examined histologically. Dilatation and curettage must also be done to exclude endometrial carcinoma.

LASER THERAPY

In 1970 *cryosurgery* (freezing of tissue) was introduced as a method of treating conditions of the cervix such as cervicitis and early cytological changes. Now the laser beam is being used in some centres for treating cervical intraepithelial neoplasia (CIN). The increase in CIN in women of childbearing age has necessitated the reappraisal of traditional treatments such as cone biopsy and hysterectomy, the laser provides a possible alternative method of treatment. Cone biopsy, involving removal of a large area of tissue results in scarring and possible interference with conception or delivery. The laser beam oblates the lesion or area effectively yet destroys little *normal* tissue, thus less scarring and stenosis of the cervix results. The long term results of laser therapy have yet to be fully evaluated. The term laser is a combination of initials from 'light amplification by stimulated emission of radiation'. The carbon dioxide laser produces a high power density beam of radiation which vaporizes tissue; because this beam is invisible a visible helium-neon laser is used simultaneously so that the CO_2

surgical beam is illuminated enabling it to be accurately directed towards the treatment site.

All lasers are potentially dangerous, the eyes in particular may be damaged by both visible and invisible radiation, the retina, cornea and lens may be irreversibly damaged. Eye protection is essential, all nurses working in laser clinics must be fully aware of the hazards of lasers and the necessary precautions which must be taken. Regular eye examination including estimations of visual acuity must be performed for all staff working with lasers. Special protective spectacles must be provided for all personnel, the one exception being the laser operator who will be performing laser surgery through the operating microscope or, in gynaecology, the colposcope.

Danger signs must be prominently displayed. A red light must be visible when the laser is in operation and an illuminated sign should read 'Laser operating'.

The patient can be treated on an outpatient basis, a general anaesthetic is unnecessary because there is little or no sensation of pain during the procedure, a paracervical block with a local anaesthetic may be used for some patients. After treatment the patient is allowed to rest for a short while before going home with instructions to return again in approximately 3 weeks. The advantages of laser treatment also include minimal haemorrhage, because the laser has a 'sealing effect' on blood vessels. Rapid healing of tissue and minimal postoperative discharge also result.

CARCINOMA OF THE UTERINE BODY

Malignant tumours of the uterus include: endometrial carcinoma—adenocarcinoma, sarcoma, and chorionepithelioma—trophoblastic disease.

Endometrial carcinoma

Unlike carcinoma of the cervix endometrial carcinoma occurs mainly in *nulliparous* or low parity women. The age group involved is commonly between 55 and 65 years. Other factors which might be associated with the disease are obesity, diabetes and hypertension. There is some evidence to support the theory that high levels of oestrogen may be responsible for some cases of endometrial carcinoma. The growth arises from the endometrium and in the early stages, because of the thickness of the myometrium, is confined to the uterine cavity (Fig. 8.8). The site of the growth is usually the upper posterior wall of the uterus.

SPREAD

Spread is by *direct invasion* of the myometrium until the growth penetrates the musculature and involves the peritoneum and/or bowel. The uterine tubes and ovaries may also be invaded. *Lymphatic* spread involves the ovarian and internal iliac lymphatic nodes and eventually the para-aortic glands. Lymphatic spread is also responsible for metastatic spread to the vaginal vault. *Blood stream* spread is

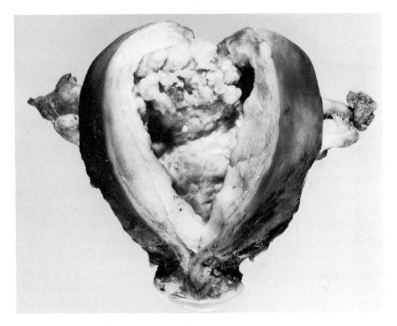

Fig. 8.8.   Carcinoma of the uterine body.

a feature of advanced disease and is responsible for metastases of the liver, lungs and brain.

CLINICAL FEATURES

The symptoms are:
> Bleeding—intermenstrual, perimenopausal or postmenopausal in this case
> Discharge—watery, blood-stained and offensive
> Pain—a late feature associated with invasion of adjacent structures

Fortunately the signs particularly intermenstrual and postmenopausal bleeding bring most patients to their doctor with early symptoms.

DIAGNOSIS

Occasionally malignant cells from the uterus may be found during routine vaginal cytology but histological examination is essential. A fractional diagnostic curettage is performed taking curettings firstly from the cervix, then the lower part of the uterus and finally the upper part. The three lots of specimen are sent in separate containers to the laboratory for microscopic examination; correct labelling of the containers is important. The naked eye appearance of curettings may make the diagnosis easier. The tissue is often friable and disintegrates when touched.

TREATMENT

The best results are said to be achieved by a combination of radiotherapy and surgery. Many gynaecologists advocate an *extended hysterectomy* (total hysterectomy with bilateral salpingo-oöphorectomy and removal of the cuff of the vagina) followed by pelvic irradiation. Others prefer to use intrauterine radium applicators prior to surgery. Occasionally radical surgery is carried out and a Wertheim's hysterectomy performed. This operation involves removal of uterus, tubes and ovaries, broad ligaments, the upper third of the vagina and also the pelvic cellular tissue and lymph nodes in some cases. The removal of the cuff of the vagina or the upper third of the vagina is performed to prevent vaginal vault recurrence, which is fairly common in carcinoma corpus.

The decision regarding treatment will be flexible and based upon the extent of the spread of the disease and the condition of the patient. In patients with advanced disease who are unfit for surgery, chemotherapy with medroxyprogesterone acetate (Provera) may induce a prolonged remission with the dosage, 100 mg orally twice daily, continued indefinitely. Radiotherapy may be used for patients who are poor surgical risks.

Sarcoma of the uterus

Uterine sarcomas are very rare representing less than 1 % of all malignancies of the female reproductive tract. Most sarcomas are highly malignant, their spread is by direct invasion and via the blood stream; the lungs are a common site for metastases. The tumour grows rapidly and results in heavy uterine bleeding, pain or ascites. The prognosis in sarcoma is poor and the patient eventually becomes cachectic.

TREATMENT

Total hysterectomy with removal of appendages may be palliative or even curative in some patients but treatment is not usually successful at the present time.

Chorionepithelioma

A rare and highly malignant tumour *chorionepithelioma* (choriocarcinoma) results in widespread metastases to the lungs or the vagina. A chorionepithelioma may follow a normal pregnancy, ectopic pregnancy or a spontaneous abortion or, as in half of the cases, a hydatidiform mole. It is a very vascular tumour which invades the myometrium and rapidly destroys normal tissue (Fig. 8.9). The tumour is dark red and fleshy, pathologically it is trophoblastic tissue which produces high

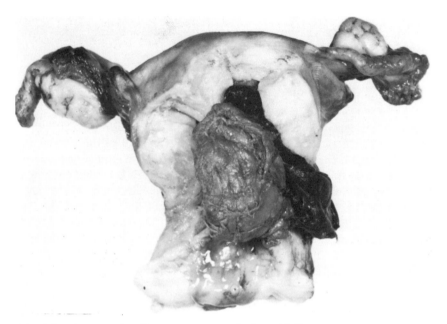

Fig. 8.9.   A rare and malignant tumour—a chorionepithelioma.

levels of human chorionic gonadatrophin (HCG). This is discovered by testing very dilute urine and finding it biologically positive of a pregnancy. Levels of HCG can be detected by blood tests also. In this case a positive pregnancy test is diagnostic of abnormal trophoblastic activity. An ultrasound scan will differentiate between a tumour or a fetus.

CLINICAL FEATURES

The symptoms are mainly heavy, irregular or continuous vaginal bleeding especially after pregnancy, abortion or hydatidiform mole. As the disease progresses other manifestations of malignant disease become obvious. Uterine enlargement, anaemia, loss of weight and signs of distant metastases become obvious. The patient may complain of chest pain and on X-ray examination of the lungs the appearance of 'puff-balls' or 'snow storm' will confirm metastatic spread.

TREATMENT

The treatment of choice is chemotherapy with methotrexate or Actinomycin D. These cytotoxic drugs have improved the prognosis of the disease remarkably, they are antagonistic to folic acid upon which the trophoblastic tissue depends heavily. Surgical treatment depends upon the patient's wishes regarding future childbearing, the extent of spread of the disease and whether or not there is per-

sistent heavy vaginal bleeding. A nurse who thoroughly understands trophoblastic disease will appreciate that a woman will suffer the same emotional
trauma as the woman who has aborted a much wanted pregnancy. Both the
patient and her husband will need support and advice for the future, and they
may feel impatient and resentful about the essential need to postpone future
pregnancies or find difficulty in coming to terms with the prospect of chemotherapy or hysterectomy (although the latter is less common nowadays since
effective chemotherapy is available).

BENIGN TUMOURS

Tumours of the uterus which are benign are endometrial polyps and fibroids.

Endometrial polyps

Endometrial polyps are small projections of the endometrium being penduncula-
ted (on a stalk). They are usually associated with endometrial hyperplasia and are
often multiple. They may be asymptomatic but may cause abnormal uterine
bleeding, or postmenopausal bleeding. Diagnosis of this condition is made by
careful exploration and curretage of the uterine cavity. Any polyps found may be
avulsed by grasping them with sponge holding forceps and twisting them
round. All material obtained must be sent for histological examination. If the
endometrial polyps recur, hysterectomy is advisable because of the risk of malignant change.

Fibroids

The correct term for a fibromyoma is *leiomyoma* (smooth muscle tumour) but
because of the fibrous appearance fibroids or myoma may be used. A *fibroid* is a
benign uterine tumour composed of smooth muscle and strands of fibrous tissue.
They are the commonest of all pelvic tumours and the incidence is thought to be
approximately 10-20 % of women over the age of 30.

The aetiology is obscure but there is thought to be a hormonal connection.
Since most fibroids atrophy after the menopause oestrogen probably promotes
their growth, this theory certainly fits the picture of endometrial hyperplasia
with which fibroids are commonly associated. There is a close association between fibroids and subfertility but nothing conclusive. Nulliparous women seem
more prone to developing fibroids.

PATHOLOGY

The fibroids' macroscopic appearance is of firm white tumours which are sometimes lobulated. Their surfaces have a whorled appearance and they have a
pseudocapsule. Microscopically interlacing bundles of muscle and fibrous tissue
can be seen. They appear to be avascular, but the pseudocapsule has blood vessels

which supply the tumour. Fibroids are commonly found to be multiple, 10-20 may be found in one uterus. They originate from seedlings but may grow to quite large sizes. Approximately 95 % of fibroids grow in the corpus, the remainder in the cervix.

All fibroids grow from small seedlings within the uterine wall. From this position they grow either inwards or outwards towards the surface of the uterus, or remain in their original positions. This growth pattern enables them to be classified as interstitial, submucous or subserous fibroids (Fig. 8.10).

INTERSTITIAL

Interstitial or intramural fibroids are situated within the myometrium. They enlarge within muscle but do not affect the uterine cavity except to increase its size. They may impair contractions of the uterus. If they are situated in the cervix they may lead to an obstructed labour.

SUBMUCOUS

Submucous or subendometrial fibroids bulge into the uterine cavity and are covered by endometrium on their outer surface. They may become pedunculated as they extrude into the uterine cavity to form fibroid polypi. This type of fibroid may become infected and give rise to haemorrhage. It may even be extruded through the cervix. These fibroids may interfere with nidation.

SUBSEROUS

Subserous or subperitoneal fibroids lie beneath the peritoneal covering of the uterus. They may 'peel' off some of the peritoneum and form a pedicle. These

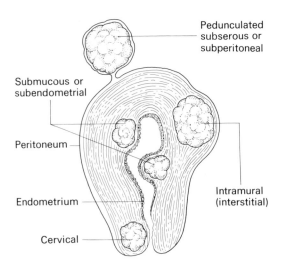

Fig. 8.10. Sites and types of fibroid.

fibroids once pedunculated may become parasitic by attaching themselves to adjacent structures or organs from which they derive their blood supply. Fibroids may also develop within the broad ligament.

DEGENERATIVE CHANGES

Fibroids may degenerate when they outgrow their blood supply which is meagre throughout. *Atrophic* degeneration occurs at the time of menstruation. *Hyaline* degeneration and necrosis occurs as a result of a poor blood supply. The cellular structure of the fibroid is lost when hyaline connective tissue replaces it. *Cystic* degeneration is preceded by hyaline degeneration. Tissue breakdown forms a fluid (liquefaction) giving the appearance of cystic spaces. *Fatty* degeneration involves patches of fatty tissue appearing in the tumour. *Calcareous* degeneration follows from calcium salts being deposited in the fatty tissue and calcification of the tumour takes place, making it visible on X-ray (often called a 'womb stone'). *Red* degeneration usually takes place during pregnancy when the fibroid undergoes necrosis. It has the appearance of red-raw meat due to the diffusion of blood pigment into the tumour. Malignant changes can take place with *sarcomatous* degeneration but the incidence is very low. Rapid enlargement of the tumour takes place causing pain and swelling from ascites.

CLINICAL FEATURES

The symptoms depend upon the size and position of the fibroid, they may in many instances be symptomless. Menstrual disturbances occur when there is an increase in the surface area of the endometrium as in submucous fibroids, endometrial hyperplasia or when uterine contractions are interfered with.

Abdominal enlargement may become obvious as the tumour enlarges. Pressure symptoms occur and the pressure may embarrass the alimentary tract causing dyspepsia and on rare occasions constipation. More usual results of pressure from the tumour are bladder disturbances such as frequency of micturition, stress incontinence and retention of urine. Urinary retention is more likely when a fibroid has become incarcerated in the pelvis. Cervical fibroids which enlarge may cause distortion of the bladder and rectum and eventually may compress a ureter. With very large tumours which might obstruct pelvic blood flow and lymphatic drainage, ankle oedema, varicose veins and haemorrhoids might be evident.

Pain is rarely experienced with fibroids unless they undergo torsion, degeneration, extrusion through the cervix or malignant change. Fibroids are associated with *subfertility* possibly blocking or obstructing the tubes by direct pressure or interfering with implantation of the fertilized ovum.

TREATMENT

Generally treatment is not necessary for women who are symptom free with a uterine enlargement of not more than the size of a 10-12 week pregnancy. The diagnosis however must be conclusive, and a diagnostic curettage may be done to rule out endometrial carcinoma. If any doubts exist as to the diagnosis, a laparotomy must be done.

SURGICAL TREATMENT

The choice of surgery will depend upon the woman's desire to have children. If a woman wishes to become pregnant and she is under 40 the operation of choice is a myomectomy. If the woman has completed her family she is advised that hysterectomy is the operation of choice, especially if she is over 40.

Myomectomy

This abdominal operation, a myomectomy, involves the 'shelling out' of the fibroids through incisions in the uterine wall. The uterus is therefore preserved for future childbearing. It is often a difficult surgical procedure and small seedling fibroids may be missed leading to a recurrence of symptoms later. It is vital to explain to the patient and her partner that if her fibroids proved too difficult to remove a hysterectomy may have to be performed. Obviously this would be a grave matter for any patient who had wished to become pregnant. Myomectomy can be a simple procedure, features which add to any difficulty are the position of the fibroids and the vascular supply.

Hysterectomy

A total hysterectomy involves removal of the body of the uterus and the cervix performed via the abdominal routes. If the fibroids are small and there is some degree of uterine prolapse a vaginal hysterectomy may be performed and an abdominal scar avoided.

NURSING CARE STUDY—MYOMECTOMY

The patient, Mrs B., was a married woman aged 34 years who had been admitted to hospital 24 hours prior to myomectomy.

Past history

In 1979, Mrs B. had a termination of pregnancy on social grounds and then in 1980 spontaneously aborted her second pregnancy. Her obstetric history is therefore para 0 + 2.

In April 1981 the patient complained of persistent right-sided pain. Laparotomy was performed and an ovarian cyst measuring 14 cm × 12 cm removed. Several fibroids were found at the operation which were thought to have caused her abortion one year earlier. Mrs B. was therefore advised to have a myomectomy before becoming pregnant again.

Medical assessment

Mrs B.'s medical assessment involved:

1 A full medical examination.
2 A pelvic examination.
3 A full blood count, haemoglobin, grouping and cross-matching.
4 An explanation of operative procedure, with the patient's written consent.
5 A prescription of premedication and night sedation as needed.

This patient was medically fit for surgery under general anaesthesia. Now a nursing plan could be prepared based on patient assessment and integrated with the medical management.

Mrs B. was a quiet rather introspective lady but seemed interested in discussing her treatment and appreciated explanations regarding planned care. She mentioned that she and her husband were concerned about future pregnancies.

It was noticed that the scar on her abdomen from previous surgery was wide, irregular and cosmetically unsightly, the surgeon intended to excise the excessive scar tissue to improve the cosmetic effect. Good nursing care must be anticipatory and potential problems must be identified (Table 8.1). In myomectomy,

Table 8.1 Myomectomy—nursing care plan.

Specific problems (potential/actual)	Objectives	Nursing action
Preoperative Patient's (and partner's) anxiety towards surgery and future pregnancies.	Lessen preoperative anxiety. Help patient (and partner) to develop a positive attitude toward future pregnancies.	Supplement doctor's explanation. Allow time for questions and discussion. Reassure about future pregnancies.
Possible guilt feelings about previous termination of pregnancy.	Help patient to come to terms with her past history. Be aware of psychological effects of a terminated pregnancy.	Allow opportunity for self-expression. Avoid confronting patient with unsolicited counsel.
Postoperative Haemorrhage from multiple uterine incisions.	Prompt recognition of signs of haemorrhage and/or reaction to blood transfusion. **NB** Check that blood grouping and cross-matching has been done prior to surgery.	Observations ½-hourly of blood pressure and pulse, colour and respirations for 6 hours. Adjust according to response and stability. Observations of vaginal blood loss.

Postoperative (continued)

Table 8.1 (continued)

Specific problems (potential/actual)	Objectives	Nursing action
		Management of established blood transfusion with routine observations.
Postoperative pain (often severe following myomectomy).	Anticipation of pain and subsequent pain relief. Be aware that pain relief may be required for a longer period of time.	Regular observations of facial expression and degree of restlessness. Direct questioning to estimate type and degree of pain. Administration of prescribed analgesia.
Urinary retention.	Promotion of urinary output. Avoidance of pressure beneath wound. Recognition of urinary retention with overflow.	Observe for distension and discomfort. Assist patient onto a warmed bedpan and support her. Run water taps and offer encouragement. Catheterization will be necessary if the above measures are unsuccessful. Record urinary output.
Abdominal distension (as a result of pelvic adhesions necessitating excessive handling of intestines).	Recognition of paralytic ileus and electrolyte imbalance.	Observe for increasing distension, nausea, vomiting, rapid pulse and absence of bowel sounds.
Circulatory stagnation (prolonged interference with pelvic blood supply).	Prevention of deep vein thrombosis.	Encourage physiotherapy, active leg movements and early mobility.

haemorrhage, adhesions and circulatory stagnation are all potential problems and so are included in the postoperative nursing plan.

Evaluation

Mrs B. made a relatively trouble free postoperative recovery. Three large submucous fibroids were removed at surgery and although haemostasis had been achieved with difficulty, no postoperative bleeding occurred. The 2 units of blood cross-matched preoperatively were given to compensate for blood loss in theatre.

There were two problems on Mrs B.'s first postoperative day: difficulty in passing urine and a febrile reaction. Actions outlined in the nursing plan helped

Mrs B. to overcome her difficulty and she soon passed large amounts of urine. A pyrexia of 38.4°C was thought to be a response to tissue trauma. She was allowed to rest and was kept pain free; a cooling fan was used and bedclothing reduced to a minimum. Oral fluids were encouraged and soluble aspirin 500 mg 4-hourly was prescribed. By evening she was apyrexial and feeling well.

The operative incision had been through the previous scar and all the redundant fibrous tissue was excised. A subcuticular suture of absorbable material closed the wound with good approximation. This much improved cosmetic effect really pleased the patient.

Mrs B. was discharged home after a stay of 8 days feeling well and optimistic about the plans for the future. Appropriate advice on coitus and pregnancy was given. (See chap. 1 on preoperative and postoperative care.)

NURSING CARE STUDY— ABDOMINAL HYSTERECTOMY

Mrs N. is a 38-year-old married woman with two children. She has been admitted to hospital following a 6 month history of 'menstrual chaos' for an abdominal hysterectomy. Mrs N. suffers from a relatively mild form of ankylosing spondylitis for which nonsteroidal anti-inflammatory drugs are prescribed. Mrs N.'s two children were both delivered by lower segment caesarean section (LSCS) because of breech presentation.

Past history

Mrs N. had been presenting with menorrhagia for 2 years and polymenorrhagia for the past 6 months. During this time a dilation and curettage (D & C) and laparoscopy was performed.

LAPAROSCOPY

A laparoscopic examination revealed several small subserous fibroids on the fundus of the uterus. The bladder was firmly stuck to the uterus.

DILATATION AND CURETTAGE

A dilatation and curettage, D & C was performed on the twenty-first day of the menstrual cycle. The histology showed irregular ripening of the endometrium, a result of insufficient production of progesterone from the corpus luteum.

Following these investigations therapy with synthetic progesterone was commenced: dydrogesterone (Duphaston) 10 mg daily from day 15 to 21 of the cycle inclusively.

Mrs N. was seen again after 6 months. There had been only marginal improvement so between the gynaecologist and the patient it was agreed that a hysterectomy had become necessary, with conservation of the ovaries.

Medical assessment

A thorough examination was carried out including full blood counts, haemoglobin 12.8 g/dl grouping (A Rh+).

Anaesthetic assessment

Particularly relevant was Mrs N.'s ankylosing spondylitis. Although relatively mild, significant points which could make a general anaesthesia hazardous would be:

Kyphosis

Limitation of chest expansion

Involvement of cervical spine

Potential problems were included in the nursing care plan (Table 8.2). Mrs N. was found to have no obvious kyphosis of her spine, her chest expansion

Table 8.2 Hysterectomy—nursing care plan

Specific problems (potential/actual)	Objectives	Nursing action
Preoperative		
Anxiety related to a fear of loss of femininity and libido/sexual function, coupled with an altered self-image.	To relieve anxiety, doubt and uncertainty. To provide insight into the condition.	Simple explanations of anatomy and physiology provide positive reassurance. Relate this to the conservation of the ovaries and the vagina.
Discomfort/pain from ankylosing spondylitis.	Ensure preoperative phase is free from discomfort and pain.	Administration of pres-cribed medication for spondylitis. Provision of adequate pillows and appliances, i.e., a fracture board placed under the mattress. Choose positions which the patient finds comfort-able during nursing procedures.
Postoperative		
Aggravation of spondylitis. Early morning skeletal pain and stiffness.	Avoidance of unnecessary strain. Prevention of postural discomfort and spinal flexion.	Prepare bed with hard base. Place patient in dorsal position on return from recovery room and whilst sleeping. Position the patient for spinal alignment and avoidance of limb hyper-flexion.

Table 8.2 (continued)

Specific problems (potential/actual)	Objectives	Nursing action
Postoperative (continued)		Give prescribed analgesia and diclofenac (Voltarol). Encourage early mobility and good posture.
Vaginal bleeding.	Early detection of vaginal bleeding PV.	Regular observations of temperature, pulse and blood pressure, colour and respiration. Vulval pad inspection at frequent intervals.
Retention.	Promotion of early postoperative voiding. Monitor urinary output and fluid intake.	Maintain intake and output chart. Assist this patient to adopt a position which facilitates voiding. Relieve any pain. Dispel anxiety by giving appropriate reassurance.
Bladder trauma (surgical dissection of bladder off uterus).	Early recognition of haematuria.	Inspection of first and subsequently voided urine for frank haematuria or less obvious smokey urine.

was good and her cervical spine was apparently unaffected. Nevertheless particular care was taken when positioning her on the theatre trolley and the table and when hyperextending her neck during anaesthetic intubation. As Mrs N. took diclofenac sodium (Voltarol) 100 mg suppositories per rectum nightly, a nonsteroidal preparation, steroid cover to avoid hypotension during surgery was unnecessary.

Summary

A total abdominal hysterectomy with conservation of both ovaries was performed. A Pfannenstiel's incision was employed, this excised previous scar tissue. The bladder which was adherent to the uterus was dissected off with some difficulty, this created a postoperative problem of urinary retention. The day after surgery Mrs N. was unable to pass urine and was therefore catherized for urinary retention. A Foley catheter remained *in situ* for 48 hours. On removal the patient was able to void spontaneously and the residual urine when measured was 100 ml. A catheter specimen of urine (CSU) revealed no bacterial growth.

Mrs N. was discharged home after 10 days and was given appropriate advice. (See chap. 1 for general preoperative and postoperative care.)

PELVIC SUPPORTS

Muscles

The structure of the muscles must be understood to fully appreciate the conditions of prolapse. It is the muscles of the pelvic floor and their neighbouring ligaments which support the pelvic organs in their proper place. The pelvic floor is formed by several muscles which either unite or overlap to form the lower boundary of the pelvic cavity. This creates a diaphragm of strong supportive muscle which is pierced in three places by the urethra, the vagina and the rectum.

The muscles of the pelvic floor (Fig. 8.11) consist of the bulbocavernosa, the perineal body, the transverse superficial perineal and the levator ani.

BULBOCAVERNOSA

The bulbocavernosa muscle encircles the vagina and runs into the perineal body. In coitus it helps contract the vaginal orifice.

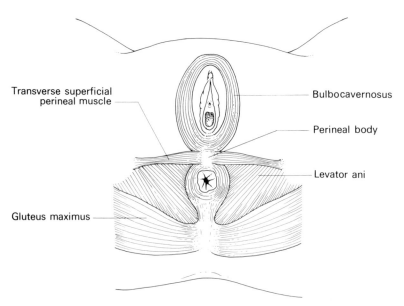

Fig. 8.11. Muscles of the pelvic floor.

PERINEAL BODY

The perineal body of muscle tissues lies between the vagina and rectum. It is vital because of the insertion of the superficial perineal and levator ani muscles. It is therefore a sort of midline sheet anchor for the other pelvic floor muscle. Its importance is emphasized when it is damaged in childbirth and the rest of the pelvic floor muscles are affected.

TRANSVERSE SUPERFICIAL PERINEAL

The transverse superficial perineal muscles run from the pubis the sacrum and pelvic side walls and are inserted into the perineal body in between the vagina and rectum. They are the least supportive of the pelvic floor muscles.

LEVATOR ANI

The levator ani muscles are the most supportive of the pelvic diaphragm. The muscles arise from the pubis, sacrum and coccyx and pelvic side walls and form a strong sheet of muscle. The fibres of these muscles are inserted into the perineal body the vagina and rectum. This insertion of fibres into the perineal body draws the muscles upwards and forwards so that a sling is formed which supports the vagina and bladder. It normally prevents a downward displacement of the contents of the female pelvis.

Ligaments

The fascia which covers the pelvic floor muscles thickens and increases in density to become the ligaments of the pelvis which fan out from the supravaginal cervix (Fig. 8.12). Most of these have been mentioned as the uterine supports, ovarian ligaments, and the infundibulopelvic ligament.

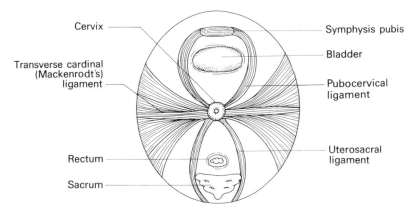

Fig. 8.12.   Ligaments of the pelvic floor.

DISPLACEMENT OF THE UTERUS

The normal position of the uterus is anteverted and anteflexed. This means that the uterus is at right angles to the vagina; it is thought that this arrangement facilitates access of the supermatazoa. Anteversion is maintained by the round ligaments and the uterosacral ligaments exert a counter positioning effect on the uterus (Fig. 8.13). On bimanual examination the fundus of the uterus is felt in the pouch of Douglas and the cervix is found to be tilting upwards towards the symphysis pubis in retroversion of the uterus.

Congenital retroversion

Approximately 15-20 % of women have a congenital (developmental) retroversion of the uterus. This does not cause any symptoms but some authorities think that a retroversion may lead to infertility. The patient's attention should not necessarily be drawn to this condition. If pregnancy does occur the retroverted uterus usually corrects itself but can become incarcerated and cause urinary retention.

Acquired retroversion

Retroversion may be caused by:
    Childbirth—puerperal retroversion
    Endometriosis—fixed retroversion
    Pelvic infection—fixed retroversion
    Tumours—fibroids
    In fixed retroversion the uterus becomes bound down by adhesions caused by previous pelvic infections.

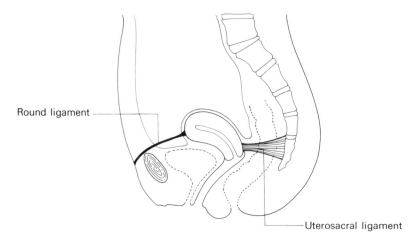

Fig. 8.13. Counter positioning effect of the pelvic ligaments.

CLINICAL FEATURES

Symptoms may include dyspareunia, dysmenorrhoea and backache. Abortion, infertility and menstrual disorders are often ascribed to a retroversion but this is of doubtful aetiology.

TREATMENT

In asymptomatic retroversion no treatment is necessary. Various pessaries are available for displacement of the uterus (Fig. 8.14). If backache or dyspareunia is troublesome the uterus may be anteverted manually and maintained in position by a Hodge pessary (Fig. 8.14b). The pessary may be left in position for approximately 6-12 weeks. If the symptoms have been relieved it can be assumed that they were caused by the retroverted position of the uterus, if the symptoms return after removal of the pessary a more permanent surgical correction will have to be considered, and this is usually the case. Whilst the pessary is in

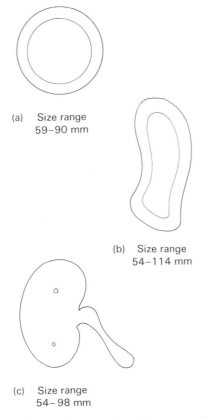

(a)   Size range
      59–90 mm

(b)   Size range
      54–114 mm

(c)   Size range
      54–98 mm

Fig. 8.14. Supportive and corrective pessaries: ring pessary (a), Hodge pessary (b), Simpsons' shelf pessary (c).

position correcting the retroversion it should not be felt by the patient, or interfere with coitus.

The basic principle of treatment is to bring the uterus forward and maintain it in this position. This is ventrosuspension and is achieved by one of the following operations, which effectively shortens the round ligament. *Gilliam's operation* consists of the loops of the round ligaments being brought through the rectus muscle and sutured together to the back of the rectus sheath on each side. *Plication of the round ligaments* involves pleats or tucks being made as a means of shortening the round ligaments.

If the retroversion is of the acquired type underlying causes such as pelvic infection or tumour must be treated.

PROLAPSE

Uterovaginal prolapse

With a uterovaginal prolapse there is a *downward* displacement of the pelvic structures. When the uterus prolapses it is invariably accompanied by descent of the vaginal walls, however the vaginal walls may prolapse without a uterine prolapse occurring. Prolapse is caused by weakening of supporting muscles and ligaments. It is mainly found in women who are parous and who have reached the menopause. Because of the muscular weakness of the pelvic floor and vagina, the adjacent pelvic structures may bulge or herniate against the vaginal walls.

CAUSES

The major cause of a prolapse is *childbearing* and the trauma which might occur during labour. During pregnancy all the muscles and supportive fascia are stretched and weakened, then during labour some of these structures are further stretched or torn. Mismanaged labour, i.e., poor judgement as to when to employ episiotomy, injudicious use of forceps and prolonged second stage of labour all lead to weakening of pelvic supports. Repeated pregnancies with only short intervals in between mean that these tissues have little chance to recover their tone.

Another cause is *congenital* or *developmental weakness* of the pelvic tissues, which may explain why some nulliparous women develop prolapse at the menopause.

A third cause is *menopausal atrophy*. Tissues deprived of oestrogen will atrophy and cease to be supportive. Prolapse in this case will only become evident at the menopause. Also women with an increased intraabdominal pressure, that is, obese women with chronic coughs, are prone to prolapse.

Vaginal prolapse

Fascial tissue closely connects the bladder and bowel to the anterior and posterior vaginal walls. If either wall prolapses it inevitably causes the adjacent organs to prolapse also.

A *cystocele* (Fig. 8.15a) is an anterior vaginal wall prolapse with herniation of the bladder. A *urethrocele* occurs if the lower portion of the vaginal wall becomes lax (see chap. 7). A *rectocele* (Fig. 8.15b) is a prolapse of the middle portion of the posterior wall of the vagina with herniation of the rectum. An *enterocele* (Fig. 8.15c) involves the upper portion of the posterior vaginal wall and the posterior fornix prolapsing which allows a loop of the bowel to herniate.

Uterine prolapse

The uterus may descend by degrees until it lies completely outside the vagina and is completely prolapsed. Three degrees are recognized:

First degree: The cervix has become elongated and descends but remains within the vagina (Fig. 8.15d).

Second degree: Further descent has taken place so that the cervix can be seen outside the introitus. It is most usually hypertrophic.

Third degree: The uterus now lies almost completely outside the introitus. In descending so far it has turned the vagina inside out. This condition is sometimes called a *procidentia* or complete prolapse (Fig. 8.16).

CLINICAL FEATURES

Features of a prolapse may be variable and it is not necessarily the large prolapse which causes the most discomfort. Common to both small and large prolapses is that symptoms are relieved when the strain from downward displacement is reduced by the patient lying down.

The main symptom which the patient complains of is 'A feeling of something coming down.' The patient also describes a sensation of dragging pain in the lower abdomen and refers to a lump 'in her front passage' or 'in between her legs'. This distressing condition may cause the patient to defer a visit to her doctor out of sheer embarrassment. Fortunately complete procidentia is relatively unusual today.

Other features include urinary symptoms, mainly difficulty in starting micturition, frequency of micturition and stress incontinence. Usually because of the prolapse position of the bladder, emptying is incomplete. Urinary tract infections are common because of urinary stasis. Defaecation difficulty may be experienced as the bowel bulges against the vagina. Also, infection of the exposed cervix may cause ulceration and vaginal discharge. Anaemia may occur if an exteriorized uterus become ulcerated and bleeds, though this is very rare. *Remember* specific questions may ascertain information not usually volunteered by the patient.

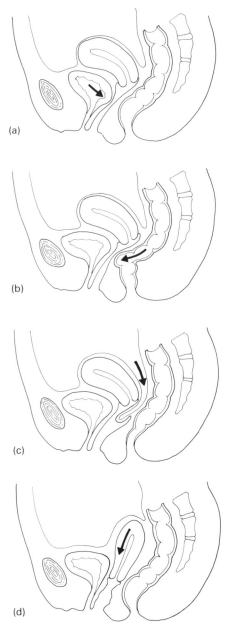

(a)

(b)

(c)

(d)

Fig. 8.15. Prolapses of the uterus: anterior wall prolapse—cystocele (a), posterior wall prolapse—rectocele (b), prolapse of the posterior fornix—enterocele (c), first degree prolapse of the uterus (d).

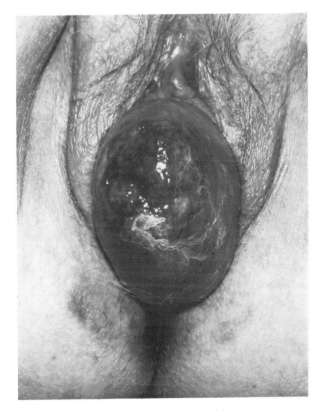

Fig. 8.16. Complete prolapse of the uterus (procidentia).

For signs of a prolapse, the patient will be examined in either the dorsal or Sims' position. In the Sims' position the anterior vaginal wall can be visualized more easily. A Sims' speculum will be used by the doctor and a cystocele easily seen when the posterior vaginal wall is retracted.

Urinary symptoms and descent of the cervix are demonstrated when the patient is asked to cough or bear down. Urine may escape from the urethra if stress incontinence is present and the cervix may be seen at the introitus.

TREATMENT

If a prolapse is found during a routine gynaecological examination and is symptomless then no treatment is required, the patient should, however, be seen and reassessed at regular intervals. If symptoms are present, treatment is usually surgical, but in patients who are physically unfit and cannot undergo surgery a supportive ring pessary may be used.

A ring pessary is particularly suitable for obese or elderly women for whom surgery would be a considerable and unnecessary risk. A Simpon's shelf pessary may be used (see Fig. 8.14c). The ring pessary is usually made of polythene or vinyl which makes it flexible. The walls of the pessary can be compressed to elongate the shape which facilitates insertion. Once a ring pessary is in position it sits firmly in the fornices and prevents uterine or vaginal wall prolapse. The patient is regularly reviewed and the ring pessary should be changed at 2-4-monthly intervals. A pessary once properly in position should not be felt by the patient.

Younger women who have not completed their family and wish to have more children may be treated by insertion of a ring pessary and seen with a view to surgery after delivery.

Two other possible lines of treatment are: pelvic floor exercises which are intended to strengthen the levator ani, and *faradism* which is the application of an electrical current to pelvic floor muscles via the vagina. Faradism is a painless treatment usually administered by a physiotherapist over a period of several weeks, pelvic floor exercises should be carried out by the patient in between applications. In these exercises the patient must be taught to tighten her buttocks and thighs several times in each hour. Through these methods muscle tone is improved and in some cases an improvement of incontinence noticed.

PREOPERATIVE TREATMENT

If surgical treatment is planned local infection of the exteriorized uterus must be treated. This may be done by 'reducing' the prolapse and packing the vagina with a length of gauze impregnated with Acriflavine cream or an oestrogen cream such as Dionoestral. Such a pack should be renewed each day until the infection subsides.

SURGICAL TREATMENT

If surgical treatment is necessary, a colporrhaphy is performed (*colp* = of vagina, *orrhaphy* = repair). A colporrhaphy involves excision of slack redundant tissue. The elevated flap of the posterior wall, e.g., the triangular shaped piece of tissue, is removed (Fig. 8.17). Whilst the vaginal wall is open underlying fascial tissue can be tightened and strengthened. When the posterior wall is open the underlying perineal body can also be repaired and reinforced.

A variety of repairs will be appropriate for each condition. For a cystocele an anterior colporrhaphy will be performed. With an urethrocele, a suburethral buttress (elevation and support of the urethra) is often combined with anterior colporrhaphy. A posterior colporrhaphy or colpoperineorrhaphy will be performed for a rectocele. A uterine prolapse will entail a Manchester operation. This is an anterior colporrhaphy, a colpoperineorrhaphy, with amputation of the cervix and tightening of Mackenrodt's and uterosacral ligaments. A vaginal hysterectomy and repair may be performed for third degree prolapse (procidentia). The nursing care plan for a colporrhaphy or colpoperineorrhaphy is outlined in Table. 8.3.

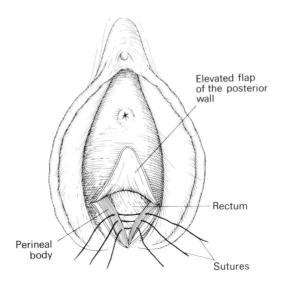

Fig. 8.17. A colporrhaphy where the elevated flap is eventually removed.

In Manchester repair (Fothergill's operation) the portion of the cervix which has usually hypertrophied and undergone first degree descent is amputated and ligaments attached to the upper vagina and supravaginal portion of the cervix (such as Mackenrodt's) are tightened. This elevates the uterus and also provides extra reinforcement to the vaginal vault, preventing enterocele later. Anterior and if indicated posterior repair are then carried out as already mentioned.

In vaginal hysterectomy the completely prolapsed uterus is removed by the vaginal route. This is then followed by the usual vaginal repair with strengthening of the vaginal vault. This type of surgery is only feasible if the uterus is not grossly enlarged or fixed by adhesions.

Table 8.3 Colporrhaphy or colpoperineorrhaphy—nursing care plan

Specific problems (potential/actual)	Objectives	Nursing action
Preoperative Urinary tract or vaginal infection.	Management of any existing infections.	Adequate fluid intake 2-3 litres/24 hours. Collection and dispatch of MSSU and HVS.
Anxiety regarding outcome and effects of surgery.	To relieve anxiety and fears of the patient (and her partner).	Explanation to the effect that sexual ability is not adversely affected and that urinary incontinence will be relieved.
Preventative care of: Trauma to the bowel (due to close proximity of the posterior vaginal wall to the bowel).	Evacuation of the bowel.	Low residue diet. Phosphate enema or bisacodyl suppositories the evening prior to the day of surgery.
Postoperative wound infection.	Vulval and perineal preparation.	Vulval and perineal ('through') shave followed by a bath.
Postoperative Discomfort from a vaginal pack.	Management of the vaginal pack.	Observation of bleeding through the vaginal pack. Check security of the pack. Removal after 24 hours.
Discomfort from an indwelling catheter.	Management of the indwelling catheter.	Catheter care: secure to thigh with strapping. Cleanse junction between urethral orifice and catheter with weak antiseptic such as chlorhexidine twice daily at least. Twice daily baths when mobilizing.
Vulval oedema, bruising and vaginal infection.	Prevention of infection and treatment of vulval swelling and/or discomfort.	Twice daily vulval swabbing with warm mild antiseptic (chlorhexidine). Application of ice packs to vulva and perineum. Application of sterile vulval pad, secured to prevent irritation.
Discomfort from perineal sutures.	Care of the perineum. Provision of optimum comfort for the patient.	Include perineal area in antiseptic swabbing. Provide patient with

NB Medical advice must be sought if gross oedema or bruising is obvious or if the perineal sutures are excessively painful.

Table 8.3 (cont.)

Specific problems (potential/actual)	Objectives	Nursing action
Postoperative (continued)		air-filled or foam ring. Remove any particularly painful suture. Assist the patient to adopt a comfortable position.
Vaginal bleeding (risk increased with amputation of cervix).	Recognition of excessive bleeding *before* and *after* removal of vaginal pack.	Frequent observation of vulval pad. **NB** A vaginal pack can obscure bleeding for a time.
Ascending infection via indwelling catheter.	Prevention of urinary tract infection. Avoidance of trauma to urethral mucosa.	Catheter care as before. Maintenance of 'closed circuit' system of drainage. Empty urinary drainage bag when two thirds full or 4-hourly. Adequate fluid intake 2-3 litres per day.
Retention of urine following removal of catheter (3-5 days).	Promotion of spontaneous voiding of adequate amounts of urine.	Instruct patient on bladder drill (see p. 86). Monitor urinary output. Measure amount of residual urine. CSU on removal of catheter.
Strain on the suture line.	To confine the bowel (initially postponing defaecation). To soften faeces.	Low residue diet. Glycerol or bisacodyl suppositories 3 days after surgery.
Constipation.	Promotion of normal bowel regimen.	Olive or arachis oil retention enema if bowels remain unopened.

NB See standard postoperative care plan for specific advice on discharge home.

9 The Uterine Tubes

Terminology may be somewhat confusing as the terms oviduct, fallopian tubes or salpinx may be used to describe the uterine tubes.

ANATOMY

The uterine tubes are oviducts (tubes along which the ova travels) which extend from the upper part of the uterus to the ovaries. They communicate with the uterine cavity and the peritoneal cavity. Each tube is composed of muscle with a lining of mucous membrane and ciliated epithelium. Their length is approximately 10 cm, and apart from their distal end they are enclosed in the broad ligament.

The uterine tubes consist of four parts. The *interstitial* or *intramural* portion lies within the thickness of the uterine muscle and has a narrow lumen. It is the shortest part of the tube. The *isthmus* extends from the uterus, it also has a narrow lumen. The *ampulla* is the widest part of the uterine tube but its lumen has numerous folds of mucous membrane, which makes it rather tortuous. The *infundibulum* is the trumpet-shaped outer end of the tube with the *fimbriae*, frond-like processes that *surround* the outer opening. This part of the tube is not covered by the broad ligament. One of the fimbriae is longer and attached to an ovary. The uterine tube is not merely a passive oviduct, it actively transports the ova along the tube until it reaches the uterine cavity. It does this by peristaltic activity of the muscular coat and by the action of the cilia.

CONDITIONS OF THE UTERINE TUBES

Diseases and disorders of the uterine tubes include acute and chronic salpingitis, pelvic inflammatory disease, ectopic pregnancy and tumours. Since the function of the uterine tube is to transport the ova from the ovary to the uterine cavity any disorder of the tubes may jeopardize future fertility. In salpingitis the infection is almost always bilateral. Tumours of the uterine tubes are exceedingly rare, most disorders are caused as a result of inflammatory disease which may also involve the ovaries, producing a salpingo-oöphoritis or a tubo-ovarian abscess.

Acute salpingitis

The causes of acute salpingitis may be postabortal infection, gonorrhoea, peritoneal infection, e.g., appendicitis, or tuberculosis. The infecting organisms in these conditions may ascend from the uterine cavity to the endosalpinx or may spread via the blood stream or result directly from a pelvic peritonitis.

In postabortal salpingitis the infection is usually due to streptococcus, staphylococcus or *E. coli*. In acute salpingitis inflammatory changes within the tube produce mucosal thickening, oedema and exudation which may leak out of the fimbrial end of the tube and cause pelvic peritonitis. In some cases exudation is trapped in the tube producing tubal distension in the shape of a chemist's retort. If the exudate is thin and watery the condition is called *hydrosalpinx*. If it is pus, the condition is called *pyosalpinx*.

CLINICAL FEATURES

The onset of symptoms may be sudden and pain is often the first symptom to occur. It may be generalized, all over the abdomen or localized in both iliac fossae. The pain is severe and bimanual examination is extremely painful for the patient. Other signs and symptoms are: malaise, nausea, pyrexia (38°C-39°C), tachycardia and purulent vaginal discharge.

The patient's abdomen may be tense, rigid and possibly distended. A pelvic mass or uterine enlargement may be felt. The leucocyte count is usually significantly raised.

TREATMENT

The patient must be admitted to hospital and nursed at bedrest until her temperature begins to subside. Preferably she should be in a single room until the results of the investigations are known. Observations of temperature and pulse must be performed 4-hourly. An adequate fluid intake should be encouraged and urinary output observed. Diet must be light and nourishing, fluids may be preferred by the patient initially.

Antibiotics are commenced once vaginal and urethral swabs are taken for gonococcal infection and blood for Wassermann reaction (WR) so that syphilis can be ruled out. Ampicillin or tetracycline is usually prescribed. Application of heat to the abdomen may give some relief, but analgesia will be required, and may initially be given intramuscularly.

Investigations will include: full blood counts, a high vaginal swab, cervical and urethral swabs and a midstream specimen of urine. Serological tests must be done if venereal disesase is suspected.

Nursing the patient in the upright position will encourage vaginal drainage, though often the patient prefers to 'curl up' in bed. All standard nursing care will be required during this acute phase, and the cause of the condition may well be an essential factor influencing the degree of psychological support which the patient may need. Vulval hygiene is vital for this patient.

A less severe type of infection may be seen in which the signs and symptoms are similar but much less pronounced. This is a subacute salpingitis and is treated in much the same way as acute salpingitis.

Chronic salpingitis

If acute salpingitis does not completely resolve, mucosal thickening and inflammation remain and a low grade infection persists. This may follow an acute attack but can occur during an acute phase. Chronic salpingitis may be caused by tuberculosis but this is comparatively rare these days.

CLINICAL FEATURES

The patient is not well, she is likely to be suffering from general malaise, lethargy and loss of appetite. Other symptoms include: dysmenorrhoea, menorrhagia, dyspareunia, vaginal discharge, and abdominal pain and backache. Most of these symptoms are intensified at the time of menstruation, or just after. There is a generalized chronic pelvic infection which may produce bladder irritability. A woman with chronic salpingitis may be infertile with tubal occlusion the cause, the fimbrial ends of each tube being fused together by adhesions. On bimanual examination tender masses are felt bilaterally and the uterus may be fixed, usually in the retroverted position.

TREATMENT

A patient suffering from chronic salpingitis may be 'run down' both physically and psychologically and will need sympathetic care. A period of bedrest is essential and analgesia must be effectively administered. Short wave diathermy may be a successful method providing local heat therapy to the pelvis, this often assists in pain relief. Antibiotics may be prescribed during an exacerbation of the condition but eventually more active management is required, and surgery becomes necessary in most cases because of chronic pelvic congestion.

In women over forty or whose family is complete a total abdominal hysterectomy should be performed. In younger women if possible ovarian tissue will be conserved. If attempts to improve the patient's fertility are intended via tubal surgery such as salpingostomy or salpingolysis, two points must be considered: the relatively low success rate and the potential risk of ectopic pregnancy.

Pelvic inflammatory disease

Pelvic inflammatory disease (PID) is an ill-defined entity but it is one of the most common diseases which affect women of childbearing age. PID is associated with salpingitis and salpingo-oöphoritis; it may occasionally be referred to as adnexitis (the adnexa is the tubes, ovaries and their mesenteries).

The aetiology of PID is that of salpingitis; predisposing factors are pregnancy, abortion and trauma. The risk is increased in women who use an intrauterine contraceptive device. *Chlamydia trachomatis* is now being associated along with other organisms as a cause of PID. It results in recurrent episodes of fever, pain and menstrual irregularities. A sticky purulent exudate may leak through the fimbriated end of a tube and settle in the pouch of Douglas (POD).

The signs and symptoms are those of acute and chronic salpingitis, which have been mentioned previously.

DIAGNOSIS

Diagnosis is based on the clinical features but exploratory techniques may provide confirmation: A *laparoscopy* will reveal inflammatory changes and fibrotic adhesions may be seen binding pelvic organs together. A *colpotomy*, that is, an incision into the posterior vaginal wall may drain purulent fluid from the POD or a tubo-ovarian abscess. A *culdocentesis* involves a needle being passed into the POD through the posterior vaginal fornix which may also promote drainage of purulent fluid.

TREATMENT

Antibiotics such as penicillin and gentamicin may be effective but as this is a recurrent condition surgical treatment eventually becomes inevitable for most women. Total abdominal hysterectomy with bilateral salpingo-oöphorectomy is performed. Ovarian tissue is conserved in younger women whenever possible.

Although PID is obviously very definitely associated with salpingitis it may be caused by an ascending pelvic infection and therefore merits this separate reference.

Ectopic pregnancy

Implantation of the fertilized ova in an extrauterine site is known as an *ectopic pregnancy*. The exact incidence is difficult to define but what seems certain is that the incidence is increasing. Ectopic pregnancies are more prevalent in developing countries.

AETIOLOGY

There may be no obvious cause found to explain the course of events, but several factors may be implicated: developmental abnormalities such as hypoplasia or extreme tortuosity of the tubes; previous tubal inflammation from acute and chronic salpingitis, or pelvic sepsis; over-development of the ovum; and, intra-uterine contraceptive devices (IUCD).

The case against IUCDs is not absolutely proven but they are thought to be causal agents, and women with an IUCD *in situ* seem to be more prone to pelvic sepsis. Also its presence may activate an otherwise dormant infection.

In over-development of the ovum, it may be that after fertilization takes place the ovum may migrate across the pelvis to enter the tube furthest away; or trophoblastic development advances too quickly, so that instead of journeying to the uterine cavity it implants in a tube. Eventually it may erode through and cause severe haemorrhage.

SITES OF IMPLANTATION

Rarely a very small percentage of ectopics may implant on an ovary, on the intestine or in the broad ligament. The ovum usually implants in the ampulla, the isthmus or the interstitial (Fig. 9.1). The reason why the ovum implants more frequently in the ampulla is that the lumen of the ampulla, despite being larger than the isthmus or interstitial portion, has a series of tortuous folds of mucus membrane through which the ovum has difficulty negotiating if adhesions or inflammation is present.

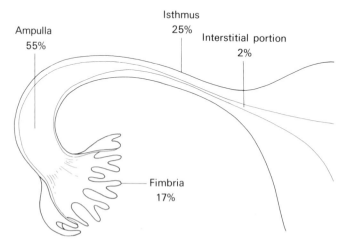

Fig. 9.1.   Sites and percentages of implantation of an ectopic pregnancy.

OUTCOME

The outcome of an ectopic pregnancy is that termination occurs at around the sixth to eighth week in one of the following ways: tubal abortion (65 % approximately), tubal rupture (35 % approximately) or tubal mole.

In a tubal mole the ovum dies but remains in the tube surrounded by old blood. This condition resembles missed abortion. Occasionally absorption of the ovum may take place prior to mole formation. In tubal abortion which is the commonest outcome of ectopic pregnancy the ovum is extruded through the fimbrial end of the tube. The tube may be able to expel all of the ovum but if expulsion is incomplete profuse intraperitoneal bleeding takes place. Blood pools in the POD and is called a pelvic haematocele (Fig. 9.2).

Very rarely the conceptus which has been expelled may survive and become a secondary abdominal pregnancy. A few of these pregnancies may survive and go to 'term'. Those that do, survive by attaching to the bowel or other abdominal structures, and deriving nourishment from them. More often the fetus will die and undergo calcification (*lithopaedion*).

A tubal rupture is the most dramatic outcome of ectopic pregnancy and occurs

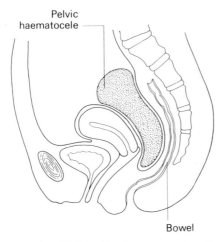

Pelvic
haematocele

Bowel

Fig. 9.2.   Pelvic haematocele with blood in the peritoneal cavity.

more usually when implantation has taken place in the isthmic or interstitial portion of the tube. The trophoblast burrows deeply into the tube which eventually ruptures. An adjacent blood vessel is usually also eroded so that haemorrhage is severe, either into the broad ligament or intraperitoneal. Haemorrhage may be sudden and massive.

CLINICAL FEATURES

The clinical signs of an ectopic pregnancy will include *amenorrhoea* (1-2 missed periods). Breast changes and uterine enlargement consistent with pregnancy may be evident. There may be acute pain, lower abdominal, as the tube distends, and bleeding begins. Vaginal bleeding, often following spasm-like pain, will be scanty and brown, and a decidual cast may be passed.

A patient admitted with a suspected ectopic pregnancy may look anxious and uneasy. If rupture has occurred she will usually display all the signs of internal bleeding namely low blood pressure and tachycardia, palor and sweating will be evident. She may have a low grade pyrexia. A rupture eventually causes *shock* and *collapse*. The classical feature of a ruptured ectopic pregnancy is the presence of shoulder tip pain. This is referred pain caused by free blood irritating the diaphragm. The abdomen may be distended and tender. Occasionally the abdomen may be rigid.

The presentation of an ectopic pregnancy is often more insidious and more difficult to diagnose, even if a rupture has taken place. Not all patients form a pelvic haematocele. Frequent (½ hourly) observations of blood pressure and pulse are necessary. A vaginal examination will be done with great care as this may precipitate a rupture, the cervix when moved will be extremely tender. The patient may not be able to *tolerate* vaginal examination.

If there is doubt about the diagnosis or an ectopic pregnancy needs to be excluded a laparoscopy may provide confirmation. A scan may reveal an empty uterus, and possibly a mass to either side.

MANAGEMENT

The admission to hospital of a patient with an ectopic pregnancy is a surgical emergency, the priorities are immediate treatment of haemorrhagic shock and pain. An intravenous infusion will be commenced immediately and blood taken for urgent cross-matching. A laparatomy will be performed at once so that the source of haemorrhage can be found and haemostasis achieved. Salpingectomy is usually performed and free blood in the peritoneum is aspirated. With a ruptured uterine tube (Fig. 9.3) there is extrusion of the conceptus. The gross disorganization of the tube makes reconstruction difficult, if attempted, coupled with the risk of a recurrent ectopic pregnancy. The remaining tube will be carefully examined. In the absence of a second tube reconstruction may be attempted if it is important to retain fertility.

Once bleeding has been arrested recovery is rapid and a potentially fatal outcome avoided. For the patient however the whole episode has been sudden and frightening and equivalent in emotional terms to any other loss of pregnancy. The nursing care plan for a patient presenting with a ruptured ectopic pregnancy is shown in Table 9.1.

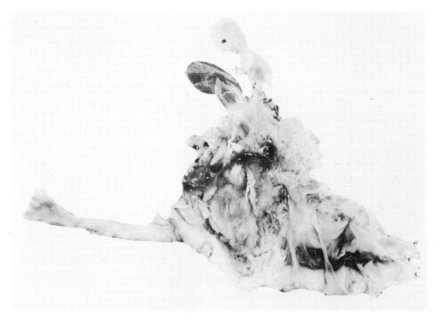

Fig. 9.3. Ruptured ectopic pregnancy.

NURSING CARE STUDY—ECTOPIC PREGNANCY

Mrs G. is a 27-year-old married West Indian woman with one child aged 3 years.

Past history

In the past Mrs G. had complained of secondary infertility and a thorough series of investigations performed. A laparoscopy revealed a suspected bilateral hydrosalpinges and evidence of peritubal adhesions. Hydrotubation demonstrated tubal patency but with very slow spillage from both tubes. A dilatation and curettage showed normal secretory endometrium. Following these investigations a salpingolysis was performed to free adhesions which had been seen on the fimbrae of both tubes.

Medical assessment

One year later Mrs G. has been admitted to hospital after being seen by her general practitioner and diagnosed as undergoing an inevitable abortion. Because of her past history the possibility of an ectopic gestation was obviously considered as an alternative diagnosis. A pregnancy test proved negative and the result of an ultrasound scan was inconclusive, therefore Mrs G. was taken to theatre for evacuation of the uterus under general anaesthesia.

Surgical treatment

Preparation for surgery included full blood count and grouping, and a sickle cell test which was negative. The possibility of an ectopic gestation was again considered as histopathological examination of uterine curettings revealed only a small amount of decidua and no trophoblastic or placental tissue. When the histology was available a further vaginal examination was carried out on Mrs G., this time it provoked acute pain therefore an urgent laparotomy was arranged. Three units of blood were cross-matched.

The situation was fully explained to Mrs G. and her husband before operative consent was obtained.

Summary

At laparotomy a ruptured gestational sac was found with blood clots and an estimated one litre of blood in the peritoneal cavity. Fortunately the right uterine tube and both ovaries appeared to be healthy. The right ovary contained a corpus luteum. Left salpingectomy and peritoneal toilet were carried out.

Table 9.1 Ruptured ectopic pregnancy—nursing care plan

Specific problems (potential/actual)	Objectives	Nursing action

Preoperative
Minimal preparation is required as surgical intervention is urgent. The patient is dressed in theatre garments and properly identified. Her consent will be obtained. *Never* **GIVE BOWEL PREPARATION, this could prove fatal. It may be necessary to aspirate gastric contents via a nasogastric tube, if fluids or a meal have been taken recently.**

Specific problems (potential/actual)	Objectives	Nursing action
Shock.	Restoration of body fluids. Resuscitation.	Management of intravenous replacement of saline/plasma/blood. Monitor vital signs, e.g., blood pressure, pulse and respirations. Nurse the patient flat and ensure quietness and warmth. Administer oxygen if dyspnoea or cyanosis become obvious. All this is done quickly as surgery to control haemorrhage is the immediate priority. Give reassurance by providing adequate explanations. Restrict oral fluids. Elevating the foot of the bed is not recommended because of the likelihood of free fluid in the abdominal cavity.
Pain can be severe and may cause shock. It can be accompanied by nausea.	Prompt pain relief with control of nausea or vomiting.	Administration of prescribed analgesia, e.g., morphia or pethidine with Perphenazine IM.
Anxiety.	Appreciation that anxiety is manifest in this condition.	To stay with the patient at all times, giving continuous support and reassurance. Involve the patient's partner here.

Table 9.1 (continued)

Specific problems (potential/actual)	Objectives	Nursing action

Postoperative

In spite of the dramatic onset and potentially devastating effect which a ruptured ectopic pregnancy has upon a woman, recovery after surgery is usually rapid and uncomplicated. A pyrexia is common in the first days. It is usually due to absorption of old blood from the peritoneal cavity.

Specific problems (potential/actual)	Objectives	Nursing action
Febrile reaction.	Detection of pyrexia and tachycardia.	Observation of temperature and pulse 4-hourly. Early encouragement to take adequate fluids. Administration of prescribed antibiotics.
Psychological effects.	Anticipation of anxiety on the part of the patient (and her partner) regarding future pregnancies.	Explain to the couple that the remaining tube is healthy and apparently patent and that tests will be arranged to confirm this.

10 The Ovaries

ANATOMY

The ovaries are homologous with the testes in the male. They are situated to either side of the uterus and are attached to the back of the broad ligament (outside the peritoneum). The ovaries are attached to the back of the uterus, just below the uterine tubes by the ovarian ligament (Fig. 10.1). They are also attached to the pelvic side walls by another ligament, the infundibulopelvic ligament. They are whitish grey in colour and have a pitted scarred surface due to the formation of previous corpora lutea. They measure approximately 3 cm × 2 cm × 1 cm.

If the ovaries are bisected they are seen to have a *cortex* and a *medulla* (Fig. 10.2). The cortex is made up of fibrous tissue and specialized cells and has an outer layer called the germinal epithelium. The medulla is made up mainly of loose connective tissue which contains blood vessels and lymph vessels. These lymphatic vessels are important in the spread of malignancy in diseases of the ovary.

At birth each ovary contains thousands of primary follicles, after puberty some of these follicles undergo development and maturation to become Graafian follicles. After ovulation the corpus luteum (yellow body) and corpus albicans (white body) are formed.

The function of the ovaries is dealt with in chapter 5. Briefly, they are involved in the production of the ova, the secretion of oestrogen and progester-

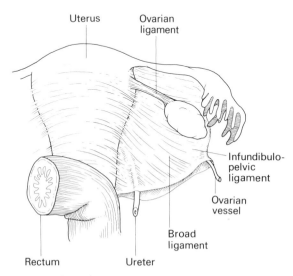

Fig. 10.1. Ligaments of the ovary.

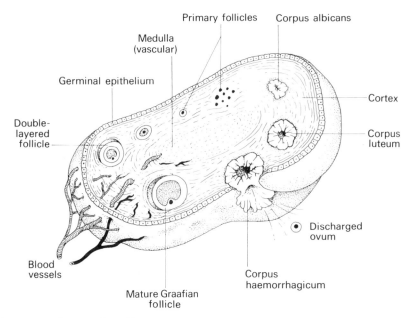

Fig. 10.2.   Cross-section of an ovary.

one, and they may also produce small quantities of androgens. Oestrogen and progesterone are hormones which control reproductive functions and are responsible for female characteristics, such as, the quality of hair and skin, and timbre of voice.

CONDITIONS OF THE OVARIES

The ovaries may develop benign cysts or malignant tumours. Many of the cysts in the benign category have a tendency to malignancy and this makes classification difficult. Oöphoritis which is an infection of the ovary seldom occurs alone. It is usually found accompanying a tubal infection (salpingitis) and is termed salpingo-oöphoritis. Occasionally a tubo-ovarian abscess may be the outcome of salpingo-oöphoritis (see p. 135).

Classification of ovarian cysts or tumours is very difficult because of their diverse nature and obscure origin. The histology of ovarian tumours can be so complex that pathological classification can be extremely difficult. This difficulty is enhanced by various hormonal changes which the ovary undergoes.

Ovarian cysts

A broad classification of ovarian cysts will include retention (distension) cysts, serous and mucinous cystadenoma, papilliferous cysts, ovarian endometrioma and dermoid cysts.

RETENTION (DISTENSION) CYSTS

Follicular and *luteal cysts* are fluid-filled, the former contain the Graafian follicle and the latter the corpus luteum. They are usually symptomless but if bleeding occurs into the cavity, especially of the luteal cyst, rupture may take place into the peritoneal cavity producing shock and symptoms similar to those of ectopic pregnancy.

SEROUS CYSTADENOMA

Single cavity cysts or *serous cystadenoma* are filled with thin straw-coloured fluid. Often the cysts are bilateral but seldom grow beyond 10-15 cm in diameter. They have a definite tendency to become malignant.

MUCINOUS CYSTADENOMA

Mucinous cystadenoma (pseudomucinous cystadenoma). These cysts are multilocular and contain a thick viscous fluid. It is a common cyst that may grow to an enormous size. Several cysts have been reported weighing 157.5 kg. Occasionally these cysts rupture and leak their contents into the peritoneum causing a condition called pseudomyxoma peritonei. A small proportion of these cysts become malignant.

PAPILLIFEROUS CYSTS

Serous cysts which are complicated by the presence of papilliferous growths (wart-like processess), grow into the cyst cavity and may eventually fill the cyst. These cysts are potentially malignant, they may erode the cyst capsule and spread to other pelvic structures.

OVARIAN ENDOMETRIOMA

Ovarian endometrioma (chocolate cysts) commonly occur in association with endometriosis. Here the cyst cavity is lined with endometrium which responds to hormonal stimuli therefore bleeding is into the cyst. Eventually the blood becomes dark and thick, hence the name chocolate cysts.

DERMOID CYSTS

Dermoid cysts (benign teratoma) derive from primordial germ cells and hence contain many different types of tissue. They are thick-walled cysts filled with sebaceous matter, hair, teeth, bone and even thyroid tissue in some cases. (Fig. 10.3). Dermoid cysts are unilocular and they can occur between the ages of 20-40.

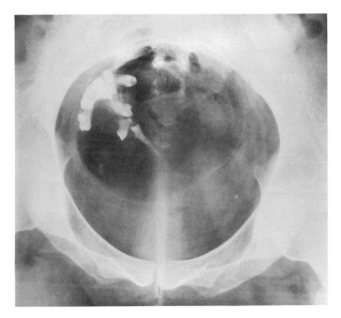

Fig. 10.3. Dermoid cyst, with teeth clearly visible.

CLINICAL FEATURES

Ovarian cysts (Fig. 10.4) can occur at any age but are most common between the ages of 35-55 years. They may be symptomless, or produce symptoms relating to the size of the cyst. *Increasing girth* is often mistaken for middle-age obesity and ignored until considerable abdominal swelling is noticed (Fig. 10.5). *Pressure symptoms* may result from pressure being exerted on adjacent structures, such as, the bladder and the gastrointestinal tract. Large tumours may cause dyspnoea, varicose veins and oedema. *Backache* is often related to the weight of the cyst. Fixation of the cyst by adhesions may cause *dyspareunia*, and *menstrual disorders* may result from hormone secreting cysts, i.e., follicular cysts. *Pain* may be caused by torsion or rupture of a cyst.

COMPLICATIONS

Complications of ovarian cysts may involve torsion or rupture of the cyst, bleeding into the cyst, malignant changes, or obstructed labour in pregnancy.

TREATMENT

Treatment is essentially surgical and the extent depends upon the age of the patient, symptoms and preference regarding future childbearing. Occasionally an ovarian biopsy may be taken via the laparoscope. If malignancy is suspected a total hysterectomy with bilateral salpingo-oöphorectomy will be performed.

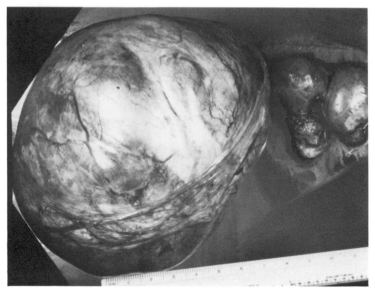

Fig. 10.4. Ovarian cyst, with uterus and ovary.

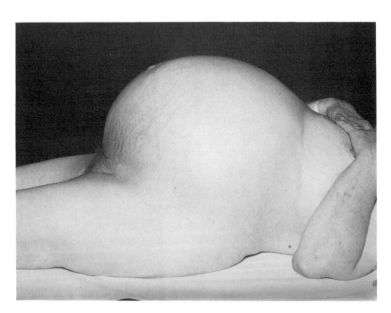

Fig. 10.5. Increased girth due to an ovarian cyst.

With simple cysts an ovarian cystectomy may be possible or otherwise an oöphorectomy.

Malignant tumours

Carcinoma of an ovary may occur at any age but is most likely after the menopause, between the ages of 45-55 years.

An ovarian carcinoma may be *primary* or *secondary*, the majority being primary, occurring as a malignant transformation in a previously benign cyst. A secondary carcinoma of the ovary may result from a primary site in the colon, bowel or breast. A rare secondary ovarian carcinoma, Krukenberg tumour may result from a primary lesion in the stomach.

Unfortunately ovarian malignancy is usually well-advanced by the time it is discovered. Secondary spread has almost inevitably taken place to the peritoneum, the lymphatic glands, and later to the liver and the lungs. In approximately 70 % of cases spread has occurred and involves both ovaries, a bilateral ovarian malignancy (Fig. 10.6). Symptoms are vague and may not be apparent in the early stages which is the tragedy of the disease.

CLINICAL FEATURES

Loss of weight, nausea, weakness and abdominal discomfort may be complained of as the disease advances. Pain is unusual. Increasing girth will be noticed by the patient and menstrual disturbance may be reported. Ascites occurs as soon as secondary spread to the peritoneum takes place and eventually the patient develops oedema of the legs, and looks pale, emaciated and very ill. On examination a hard mass can be felt in the abdomen.

The patient is in a very distressed condition as respiratory and gastrointestinal function is embarassed by gross abdominal distension. The prognosis for ovarian malignancy is generally poor.

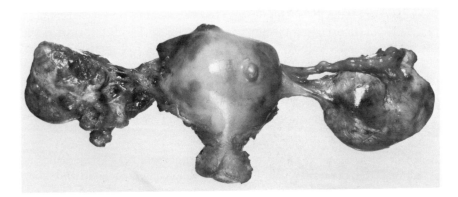

Fig. 10.6. Bilateral malignant ovaries.

TREATMENT

Most cases of ovarian carcinoma require a laparotomy to determine the exact degree of spread. Most surgeons will attempt to resect as much of the malignant tissue as possible, a bilateral salpingo-oöphorectomy and a total hysterectomy plus an omentectomy being performed if possible. Even if this fairly radical surgery proves unsuccessful in the long term, the patient will have been relieved of some of the distressing pressure symptoms in the meantime.

Radiotherapy

Radiotherapy may be used to confine the disease or as an adjuvant to surgical treatment. Megavoltage dosage may produce distressing side effects.

Chemotherapy

Chemotherapy has been used in the past, mainly to modify the effects of ovarian malignancy, often as an adjuvant to radiotherapy or surgery. Occasionally an intraperitoneal instillation of a cytotoxic drug such as cyclophosphamide may be used at the time of surgery, though this is now less common.

Significant advances have been made in chemotherapy with cytotoxic drugs and there has been an increase in the number of women surviving for up to 2 years or beyond. The introduction of several new cytotoxic drugs is largely responsible for this improvement in treatment with chemotherapy. These new drugs which include agents such as vinblastin, bleomycin and more recently cisplatin are used in combination with each other so that different factors within cancer cells can be attacked. Various schedules can be used each made up of a different combination of cytotoxic drugs. Therapy is 'pulsed' so that drug-free periods allow normal tissue to recover. Even though cytotoxic therapy may not be curative, in many instances a palliative effect will be achieved which usually improves the quality of life in the survival time.

As cytotoxic drugs are extremely toxic and affect normal as well as malignant tissue, frequent and regular monitoring of the leucocyte and the platelet counts is necessary. If cytotoxic drug therapy produces extreme side-effects, such as persistent nausea and vomiting, its continued use in the treatment of advanced ovarian cancer may not be justified. The nursing care of patients with advanced ovarian cancer must be highly skilled and sympathetic, managing both physical and psychological aspects of the disease is essential.

NURSING CARE

A patient in the terminal stages of carcinoma ovary will need sympathetic and skilful care from the ward team. The doctor, nurse, physiotherapist and others must work together to ensure that the patient spends her remaining time in comfort and tranquillity, that pain or discomfort is minimal and that adequate rest and sleep is possible. A nursing care plan is shown in Table 10.1. The patient will benefit physically and psychologically if she is encouraged and helped to remain active for as long as possible.

In the final stages of the disease the woman will be very much aware that despite treatment she is not getting better. She is aware that although her abdomen is getting larger the rest of her body is wasting away. She will feel weak and unwell. This woman must be allowed to express her feelings and talk freely about her fears and uncertainties. Medical and nursing staff must respond to this patient's questions sensibly so that uncertainty is lessened and support provided during the period in which she attempts to come to terms with her condition. Relatives and close friends should be included at this time so that they too can offer the much-needed support, and indeed derive some comfort themselves. Spiritual needs of the woman and her family may be provided by the clergy.

Paracentesis abdominis

Tapping of ascites from the peritoneal cavity by paracentesis abdominis, so that abdominal pressure may be relieved, is done at necessary intervals. The patient obtains relief from this procedure and this must be explained to her. Principles of asepsis must be maintained throughout this procedure. The procedure involves:

1 The patient is comfortably positioned either sitting upright or semirecumbent in her bed after first emptying her bladder.
2 The trocar and cannula is then inserted to the left or right of the abdominal midline. (A local anaesthetic makes this less painful for the patient and a scalpel may be used to nick the skin.)
3 The trocar is removed and the tubing attached to the cannula which remains *in situ*. The length of tubing is then connected to a drainage bag hanging in a dependant position.
4 The trocar can be secured to the abdomen with a guaze swab and some strapping. A supportive binder may be applied for comfort, and support.
5 A screw clip may be placed on the drainage tubing so that drainage can be controlled, too rapid a removal often produces an unpleasant sensation with the intraabdominal pressure reduced too suddenly.
6 The drainage bag must be emptied at regular intervals and the amount of drainage charted.
7 The site of the paracentesis must be inspected regularly and re-dressed if necessary.

Once fluid drainage has been established the nurse must make the patient comfortable, offer her a drink and allow her to rest. Some extra reassurance at this stage will be appreciated by the patient who may have found the procedure rather alarming and uncomfortable. The pulse rate must be observed at regular intervals.

Table 10.1 Terminal ovarian malignancy—nursing care plan.

Specific problems	Nursing action

The nurse will be fully aware of the terminal nature of this disease and allow for modifications in care which will cater for needs of both mind and body. The patient's condition must be continually reassessed so that nursing care can be reviewed in line with any changes and any appropriate modifications made.

Specific problems	Nursing action
Psychological stress: fear, anxiety, depression.	Assist the patient to come to terms with the future by answering her questions; provide explanations which will suit *this* particular woman. *Offer* the *truth*, the patient will often develop her own individual way of coping with the situation. *She* may even choose not to refer to the matter again, and use her own coping mechanisms. (A junior nurse would be well advised to seek advice from a senior nursing colleague on this issue.) Administration of prescribed preparations which might induce a feeling of well being, i.e., elixirs containing morphine.
Loss of appetite and/or reduced fluid intake.	Attempt to stimulate an interest in food and fluids. Offer *small* portions of attractively served foods which the patient would like. Respect the patient's preference regarding types of food, chilling of liquids etc. Before serving food and fluids give mouth care as necessary. An appetite stimulant may be helpful, such as a small glass of sherry or prescribed tonic.

Table 10.1 (cont.)

Specific problems	Nursing action
Resulting from pressure:	
Abdominal distension: ascites.	Nursing management of paracentesis abdominis involves positioning the patient upright so that continuous drainage is facilitated. Re-apply abdominal binder so that counter-pressure relieves discomfort.
Abdominal discomfort or pain.	Sensible administration of prescribed analgesia so that pain may be anticipated. Adaptation of positional change.
Gastrointestinal upset: nausea, vomiting, indigestion and constipation.	Constipation may cause nausea and vomiting. Fibre in the diet and the use of preparations which add bulk to stools may be helpful. Fluid intake must be adequate. Antiemetics may be necessary.
Respiratory embarrassment.	Nurse the patient upright or sitting in a chair for as long as possible. Relief of ascites usually improves breathlessness.
Oedema	Elevate and protect oedematous limbs from pressure by use of appliances, e.g., bed cradles.
Associated with weight loss:	
Pressure sores and loss of integrity of the skin.	Maintain *gentle* mobilization for as long as possible to allow optimum perfusion of vital organs and tissues. Attend to hygiene. Use of sheep skins, bed cradles, etc. whilst in bed.
Weakness, lassitude.	Modify nursing care as deterioration becomes obvious.

Rare ovarian tumours

Granulosa cell tumour, arrhenoblastoma, dysgerminoma, Brenner tumour and fibroma are rare and are only discussed very briefly. These are mainly hormone-secreting tumours and the treatment is essentially surgical.

GRANULOSA CELL TUMOUR

Granulosa cell tumours are composed of similar cellular tissue to that of the Graafian follicle. Like the Graafian follicle they produce oestrogen and due to the excessive production of oestrogen feminization is obvious. Precocious menstruation, hypertrophy of breast tissue and external genitalia may be seen in puberty but in older women the effects are mainly on the menstrual cycle. In postmenopausal women, bleeding is the most obvious sign. Approximately 25% of these tumours may be malignant.

ARRHENOBLASTOMA

An arrhenoblastoma is an extremely rare tumour which has a masculinizing effect. It may cause amenorrhoea, hirsutism, atrophy of the breasts and deepening of the voice. These effects are caused by the tumour secreting testosterone. These tumours are potentially malignant.

DYSGERMINOMA

A dysgerminoma tumour is most often seen in children and young women. It secretes neither male or female hormones. It is often found to be malignant, but is very radiosensitive.

BRENNER TUMOUR

A small tumour comprising of fibrous tissue, the Brenner tumour, occurs mainly in postmenopausal women.

FIBROMA

A benign neoplasm which arises from the ovarian cortex is known as a fibroma. It may be a small nodular growth or larger, sometimes appearing to replace the ovary. Although this tumour is benign it may occasionally be associated with ascites and hydrothorax, this is known as *Meigs' syndrome.*

11 Sexually Transmitted Diseases and Pelvic Infection

SEXUALLY TRANSMITTED DISEASES

In 1961 a statutory classification of venereal disease (VD) was made by the UK Government. This included gonorrhoea, syphilis and chancroid, other diseases which are transmitted by sexual contact and also nonspecific genital infections. These form a formidable list, included are: pediculosis pubis (pubic louse), genital scabies, herpes simplex, genital warts, candidiasis, trichomoniasis and chlamydia. Two diseases which are more common in tropical countries are lymphogranuloma venereum (LGV) and granuloma inguinale.

Reports from the World Health Organisation (WHO) state that VD is increasing worldwide despite other infections declining. In 1971 the International Union against the Venereal Disease and Treponematoses (IUVDT) investigated the tremendous increase in the incidence of sexually transmitted diseases (STD) in the USA. Obviously understanding of and attitudes towards STD require reappraisal. Widespread public education appears ineffectual in changing attitudes towards sexual behaviour.

Other factors which appear to be partly responsible for the upsurge are the nonprotective forms of contraception such as the 'pill' and IUCD. The use of the condom, now less popular than in the past did offer some protection from disease, for both partners.

The media also must accept some responsibility for 'over-promoting' sex. It is little wonder that young people attempt to become sexually experienced premaritally when, from the way sex is 'hyped' by the media, it is clearly something to experience, even if a relationship is transient. New evidence, however, seems to suggest that the age group 20 plus is more promiscuous than the 16-20s. Within this section on STD, gonorrhoea, syphilis, chancroid, nonspecific genital infections, warts, infestations, herpes genitalis, *Candida albicans* and *Trichomonas vaginalis* are considered.

Gonorrhoea

Gonorrhoea is the most common of the venereal diseases, it is also the easiest *treatable* infection in the world. In 1879 Albert Neisser isolated the bacterium of gonorrhoea hence the name *Neisseria gonorrhoeae*. It may infect male or female, old or young, heterosexual or homosexual. Despite effective worldwide treatment there is no diminution of this disease, and resistant strains are creating even greater problems.

Gonorrhoea is difficult to detect in women since it may be completely asymptomatic and even when symptoms are present they are rather vague. Frequency and dysuria may be a mild problem. Vaginal and urethral discharge may present but the woman herself may relate this to normal vulval moistness. Even when the vaginal discharge becomes thick and yellow the condition may be overlooked. This lack of specific symptoms is one of the reasons why continuing high levels of gonorrhoea remain in the community.

As the organism ascends the genital tract it may cause bartholinitis, infection of the Skene's glands and cervicitis, and eventually the uterine tubes are involved and acute salpingitis results. A gonococcal salpingitis produces acute pain in the iliac fossa, and causes menorrhagia, nausea and vomiting. Reflux of the menstrual fluid may spread the infection to the pelvic cavity causing peritonitis. Pelvic inflammatory disease (PID) is a serious complication of gonorrhoea. Eventually fibrous adhesions block the tubes and infertility or ectopic pregnancy may result. Very rarely more severe complications such as myocarditis, pericarditis or endocarditis may occur, if the disease becomes blood borne.

DIAGNOSIS

The gonococcus is difficult to detect with microscopy alone, cultures are needed. Specimens should be taken from the Bartholin's gland and the cervix and also from the urethra and the Skene's ducts by a 'milking' technique if necessary. The fixed specimens should be clearly labelled with the patient's name and the site from which the specimen was taken. If delay in transportation of the specimens to the laboratory is anticipated Stuart's transport media should be used. The technique used is to collect secretions with a special stick swab, then plunge the stick into the bottle containing Stuart's medium, the stick is then snapped off and the cap screwed on tightly.

Since patients may have more than one STD serological tests for syphilis should be done before antibiotics are prescribed.

TREATMENT

Although it appears that the gonococcus is developing some resistance to penicillin it is still the treatment of choice in gonorrhoea. Most patients can be treated as outpatients but occasionally hospitalization is necessary if serious complications such as salpingitis occur.

Procaine penicillin is administered, 4.8 g IM as a single dosage which may be repeated. Probenecid is given simultaneously to prevent excretion of penicillin. It is vital to advise the patient to avoid sexual intercourse until the infection has been treated, and to establish a means of contact tracing.

Gonorrhoea can infect the eyes of infants causing ophthalmia neonatorum ('Sticky' eye), impaired vision or blindness.

There is some evidence to support screening of *all* antenatal patients for gonorrhoea, especially unmarried mothers, since gonorrhoea *and* syphilis may coexist in one woman.

Syphilis

Fortunately, syphilis is a much less common disease than gonorrhoea but present day statistics show a worrying increase in its incidence.

The spirochaetes of syphilis, *Treponema pallidum*, enter the body through cracks or abrasions in the skin, usually during sexual intercourse. The incubation period is variable but the organism is capable of doubling its number approximately every 30 hours. Syphilis is more often found in homosexual males and prostitutes.

The first sign of syphilis in women is a soft painless lesion (*chancre*) on the vulva or mouth. Occasionally the chancre is on the cervix and not seen. A chancre appears after an incubation period of between 21 days and 90 days. This is the first stage of the disease—*primary syphilis.*

During *secondary syphilis* the disease invades the blood stream producing a generalized infection. There may be a reddish brown rash on the patient's skin which may appear on the face, trunk and limbs but which is usually symmetrical in its distribution. The patient may have a sore throat and mouth, hoarseness, and lymphadenitis or lymphadenopathy. A woman may see a gynaecologist because she has noticed wart-like growths on the vulva and perineum. These are flattened, moist epithelial thickenings called condylomata lata. These lesions teem with treponema. The patient is generally unwell and occasionally syphilitic alopecia may be seen. Syphilis in this secondary stage is very contagious and can last for up to 2 years.

Fortunately, nowadays, the disease is usually diagnosed and treated in the early stages and thus the third stage (*tertiary syphilis*) is prevented. If this late stage of the disease is reached, neurological and cardiovascular complications are severe. Degenerative changes may take place in bones and joints which eventually may cripple the sufferer. This is extremely rare in the UK.

Since *Treponema pallidum* can pass through the maternal circulation to the placenta, an infected mother could infect the fetus. All antenatal patients therefore must be routinely screened for syphilis. Thankfully congenital syphilis is very rare today.

DIAGNOSIS

The diagnosis of syphilis is made by detecting the spirochaetes. In the early stages of the disease a chancre may be scraped and the exudate examined microscopically for treponema. Later serological tests will be done such as Wassermann reaction (WR) and the Veneral Disease Research Laboratory test (VDRL). Specific tests for syphilis include: the *Treponema pallidum* immobilization test (TPI) and the fluorescent treponemal antibody absorption test (FTA ABS). Work is being done to perfect a relatively quick and simple serological test for syphilis. This is an enzyme-linked immunosorbent assay (ELISA).

Sexual intercourse should not take place until the diagnosis is certain and treatment has been completed.

Penicillin remains the treatment of choice but alternative antibiotics are available such as the tetracyclines. Deep intramuscular injections into the buttocks are necessary—dosage 1.2 g IM daily for 10-14 days.

Chancroid

Chancroid or soft sore is a highly contagious condition caused by *Haemophilus ducreyi*, a gram-negative bacillus. Males are more likely to develop a chancroid than females and it is relatively uncommon in the UK. Apparently the incidence of chancroid increased in the USA following the Vietnam War.

Initially the lesions commence as small papules on the labia and vestibular region, the perineum may be involved. These lesions eventually become painful, soft-based ulcers, which may suppurate. Inguinal lymph glands may become swollen (*bubo*) and the whole of the vulva is extremely tender.

DIAGNOSIS

The appearance of soft sores points strongly to chancroid but cultures will be taken of exudate from the ulcers to confirm the diagnosis.

TREATMENT

Any local treatments carried out on the vulval area, such as vulval swabbings, must be done with great care because of the painful nature of the condition. Bedrest and adequate pain relief will be necessary in severe cases.

The sulphonamides are usually the most effective drug treatment. Streptomycin may also be prescribed.

Nonspecific genital infections

Many genital infections are nonspecific in that the aetiology is vague because no one specific organism has been isolated. Nonspecific urethritis (NSU) and nongonococcal urethritis (NGU) are in this category of nonspecific genital infections (NSGI). The many possible causes include:

Infections:
  Bacterial, i.e., *E. coli*, chlamydia
  Protozoal, i.e., *Trichomonas vaginalis*
  Fungal, i.e., *Candida albicans*
  Viral, i.e., herpes simplex II
  Chemicals, i.e., vaginal deodorants

Apart from an NSGI which has been caused by a chemical agent or physical agent (foreign body) it is nearly always sexually-transmitted. In women NSU is not uncommon but it is a difficult condition to treat and because it recurs time and again it is important to provide adequate psychological support. Patients with NSU are likely to become depressed and despairing of a cure after years of discomfort and anxiety. Treatment is usually with tetracycline and abstinence from coitus is advisable during therapy.

Recently much more attention has been focused on a bacterium called *Chlamydia trachomatis* which appears to be implicated in up to 50 % of cases of NSU and NGU. Chlamydia is a tiny organism which is pathogenic within body cells. It is thought to be at least as common as gonorrhoea and may be a major cause of salpingitis. It is also thought to be a possible cause of cervicitis, cystitis, PID and abortion.

Warts

Like common warts, genital warts (condylomata acuminata) are caused by a virus. (See figure 6.3.) They are almost always sexually transmitted. Often these warts are unnoticed until the woman attends for gynaecological examination. Genital warts seem to flourish in moist areas and a vaginal discharge is often seen in this same patient. Proliferation of genital warts occurs during pregnancy.

Treatment is by a local application of caustic preparations such as trichloro-acetic acid or antimitotic substances, such as Podophyllin paint. Treatment should include treatment of the vaginal discharge as well.

Infestations

Phthirus pubis (pubic crab louse) and *Sarcoptes scabiei* (scabies) are both sexually transmitted infestations although prolonged contact in a warm environment may assist transmission. Treatment is by local application of benzyl benzoate or crotamiton (Eurax).

Herpes genitalis

Genital herpes is an acute inflammatory disease which is caused by herpes simplex II. It is a most distressing condition which as well as being physically harrowing is also psychologically devastating. This kind of STD is becoming increasingly more common and in the USA is reaching almost epidemic proportions.

Herpes is a recurrent disease and women can sometimes anticipate an exacerbation. The clinical signs are mainly fluid-filled vesicles on the genitalia which are extremely painful. A burning sensation is felt on micturition and frequency may be experienced. Lymph glands in the groin may be enlarged. Occasionally acute retention may result from severe dysuria. Applications of anaesthetic ointments to the vulva may be soothing and warm baths may relieve dysuria or retention though occasionally catheterization may be necessary.

Herpes genitalis is being studied much more closely today since it had definitely been implicated as possible aetiological factor in some cases of cervical intraepithelial neoplasia. In fact the cervix may be a site of herpetic lesions. This implies that certain types of cervical malignancy *may* be sexually transmitted.

Another devastating effect of herpes genitalis is upon the newborn. As the baby is delivered through an infected genital tract the infection is passed from mother to baby, because the infection may be serious and possibly fatal an elective caesarian section should be performed.

Unfortunately herpes is incurable and even though the condition clears up the virus lives on in the body so that repeated recurrence is suffered. The patient should be warned about the relapsing nature of herpes.

At present treatment consists of applying antiviral ointments such as acyclovir or solutions containing idoxuridine for 3-4 days as soon as lesions appear. The use of the laser beam may prove to be beneficial in the not too distant future. Clinical trials of a glycoprotein vaccine are at present being undertaken and it may be that vaccination will be the key to future treatment of the herpes virus.

Candida albicans and *Trichomonas vaginalis*

Both *Candida albicans* and *Trichomonas vaginalis* may be sexually transmitted. Vaginal discharge vaginitis and vulvitis may result from these infections. Candidia and trichomoniasis are mentioned in chapter 3.

SPECIAL CLINICS

In 1972, WHO said in their report that: 'The failure to control venereal disease is arousing worldwide concern.' A fundamental of control is the availability of adequate facilities and staff. In 1974 the Department of Health and Social Security issued a comprehensive booklet of guidelines for 'special' clinics, it was very detailed in every respect but the main principles which each clinic should operate to were:
1 Treatment must be provided by a specialist.
2 Treatment must be free.
3 Open access.
4 Confidentiality.
5 International cooperation.

It was suggested that clinics should be integrated with the general outpatient department rather than functioning in isolation as they have in the past. Euphemistic names for clinics seem to be disappearing and the more accurate title of Genitourinary Clinic is becoming more common. A stigma is still attached to VD despite the fact that by far the greater proportion of people who attend clinic have a STD rather than VD as statutorily defined. Referring to the specialty as genitourinary medicine may help to remove this stigma.

Attitudes of all staff working in such a clinic are particularly important. The patient may be put off by a brusque judgemental approach, and being asked personal details in an insensitive way will not help. Many patients prefer to be called by number rather than name and although the patient's wishes must be respected to the full, accurate details must be obtained so that records can be maintained.

PELVIC INFECTION

Endometritis, pelvic tuberculosis and endometriosis come within the category of pelvic infection. The differential diagnosis to endometriosis is chronic pelvic inflammatory disease (PID) which is covered in chapter 9.

Endometritis

Inflammation of the endometrium, *endometritis*, is an uncommon condition, basically because during the reproductive years the endometrium is constantly being renewed and does not allow an infection to become established. Also the vagina and cervix provide a defence mechanism against pathogens. These are disturbed after abortion or delivery. Criminal abortion is more likely to produce endometritis as are missed abortion, retained products of conception or an intrauterine contraceptive device. After the menopause when reproductive tissue becomes atrophic and the vaginal pH is alkaline little resistance to bacteria is encountered so that senile endometritis may occur.

Causative organisms include: *Streptococcus faecalis, Escherichia coli, Staphylococcus pyogenes,* gonococcal infections, tuberculosis, chlamydia.

CLINICAL FEATURES

The patient is not well and will complain of malaise and anorexia. Pain varies from low backache to pelvic pain, the temperature and pulse may be raised. The tongue is often furred. Endometritis may cause a blood-stained or purulent discharge, but if pus remains in the uterus (*pyometra*) there is gradual uterine enlargement.

TREATMENT

The patient needs to be admitted to hospital and nursed on bedrest. Antibiotics will be prescribed. Sometimes with a pyometra drainage is necessary, the cervix is dilated and a gentle curettage performed. Perforation is a danger during curettage because the infected tissues are friable. Histological examination will determine the cause of the infection. Hysterectomy may be necessary in chronic endometritis.

Pelvic tuberculosis

Tubercle bacilli are thought to be carried from a primary site, usually the lungs, to the female genital organs mainly by the blood stream. The disease usually affects younger women, the commonest site of infection being the uterine tubes,

tuberculosis salpingitis. Other sites of infection are the endometrium, tuberculous endometritis and the pelvic peritoneum, tuberculous peritonitis.

Many cases of tuberculous endometritis are discovered during investigation of
infertility when the curettings from the uterus reveal tubercle bacilli and the
uterine tubes are usually found to be blocked or distorted. Genital tuberculosis is
a common disease and should be suspected in young women complaining of
infertility, amenorrhoea or displaying symptoms of pelvic infection.

TREATMENT

Antituberculous chemotherapy is the treatment of choice. Surgical treatment is
usually reserved for those patients who do not respond to chemotherapy and consists of total hysterectomy with removal of both uterine tubes. The ovaries may
be conserved in young women.

Endometriosis

Endometriosis is a condition in which fragments of endometrial tissue or cells are
deposited in sites other than the lining of the uterine cavity. These fragments respond to hormonal stimuli, therefore when menstruation takes place they also
bleed. As there is no outlet for the blood flow it becomes trapped within a thin
stroma. Some of the blood serum is absorbed but a thick tarry residue remains,
hence the name 'chocolate cysts' (see chap. 10). When this occurs outside the
uterine cavity it is called *external* endometriosis (Figs. 11.1 & 11.2). *Internal*
endometriosis occurs when endometrial cells from the basal layer infiltrate the
myometrium causing a generalized enlargement of the uterus. More commonly
this condition is called *adenomyosis*.

Spillage of altered blood from chocolate cysts may cause dense fibrous adhesions which may incarcerate the uterus, the bowel and other pelvic structures
resulting in what is known as a 'frozen pelvis'. The uterus is usually retroverted
and retroflexed.

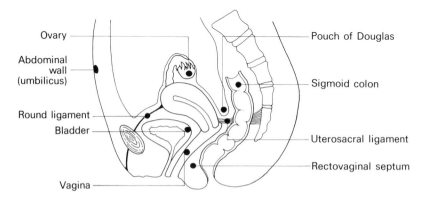

Fig. 11.1. Endometrial tissue deposited on the ovaries, uterosacral ligaments and the
pouch of Douglas.

As endometriosis is under the influence of hormones it never occurs before puberty, and after the menopause tends to regress. Nulliparous women or women who marry late and limit their family are more likely to suffer from this condition. It is found to be more common in sophisticated societies and rare in Africa or the West Indies.

CAUSES

Several theories exist as to the cause of endometriosis but the precise cause in an individual case may remain uncertain. These theories include:

1 Retrograde spillage of endometrial tissue through the uterine tubes.
2 Serosal metaplasia which suggests that peritoneal endothelial cells may undergo change and become endometrial tissue.
3 Vascular or lymphatic transport of endometrial fragments.
4 Implantation may occur when the uterine cavity is opened during surgery.

In retrograde spillage, endometrial tissue is most likely to deposit on the ovaries, uterosacral ligaments and the pouch of Douglas. Other sites of implantation are also shown in figure 11.1 but bizarre sites such as an abdominal scar or a limb have been known. Theory number 3 could explain this phenomenon.

CLINICAL FEATURES

Endometriosis may be asymptomatic in approximately 25 % of cases, in the remainder of patients pain is the outstanding symptom. *Pain* may be due to: *secondary congestive dysmenorrhoea* preceding and during menstruation; *dyspareunia* if

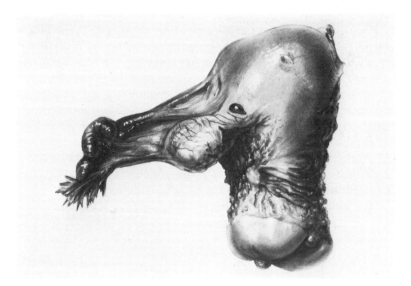

Fig. 11.2. External endometriosis.

there is fixed retroversion of the uterus caused by adhesions; involvement of the pouch of Douglas and rectovaginal septum causing pain on defaecation.

Menstrual disturbances may involve menorrhagia due to pelvic congestion, especially with uterine adenomyosis; or irregular bleeding, due to hormonal imbalance, probably caused by affected ovaries.

Infertility is a common problem and may be due to pathological disturbances of the ovary. Despite the formation of adhesions infertility is not due to blockage of the tubes but can be caused by distortion of the tubes.

TREATMENT

As with many gynaecological conditions treatment depends upon the age of the patient, her wishes regarding childbearing and her personal preference. Endometrosis is a benign condition which appears to improve or even disappear in pregnancy and which definitely regresses at the menopause. A laparoscopic examination may be helpful in determining the extent of the condition.

Hormone therapy

Hormone therapy is used to produce decidual changes in the endometrium by the creation of a pseudopregnancy. Combined oestrogen and progesterone preparations will be given to achieve this effect. Danazol (Danol) may also be prescribed. This drug inhibits gonadotrophin secretion so that ovulation and menstruation do not occur. Treatment with all types of drugs needs to be long term, at least 6-9 months duration. Side effects from hormonal treatment may force discontinuation if nausea, fluid retention or other side effects become troublesome.

Hormonal therapy is given in increasing doses so as to deliberately achieve amenorrhoea. This fact must be explained to the patient so that absence of menstruation does not alarm her, and that she understands it is an essential effect of treatment. Without stressing the negative aspects of hormone therapy unduly it is nevertheless important to warn the patient that she may feel nauseated at the outset of treatment, and may experience weight gain due to fluid retention.

Patients with deposits in the rectovaginal septum and those with adhesions usually require surgical treatment. This may be *conservative*, i.e., excision of endometrial deposits, division of adhesions and anteversion of the uterus (ventrosuspension) or *radical* when a total hysterectomy and bilateral salpingo-oöphorectomy is performed as a last resort. The extent of surgery will vary with each patient and the extent of the disease.

12 Abortion

Abortion or *miscarriage* may be defined as the expulsion of the fetus from the uterus before it is viable, i.e., before it is capable of independent existence. In law this is before the twenty-eighth week of pregnancy. An abortion may be spontaneous or induced (Fig. 12.1).

SPONTANEOUS ABORTION

Approximately 15 % of pregnancies end in abortion and most spontaneous abortions occur between the eighth and twelfth week when the corpus luteum is degenerating and progesterone secretion is reduced.

Causes

The cause of a spontaneous abortion may never be found but many factors are thought to be responsible. These may be fetal or maternal. *Fetal* factors include defects in the ova, fetus, trophoblastic tissue or placenta. There may be chromosomal abnormalities, fetal malformations or infections such as rubella.

Maternal factors concerned may include: *uterine abnormalities* which can be congenital or acquired, i.e., subseptate uterus, fibromyomata or fixed retroversion, incompetent cervix. Maternal *illness* involving a general systemic disease, e.g., diabetes, acute infection, chronic nephritis, may affect the fetus as would thyroid disease. Syphilis may cause a late abortion, or a still birth. *Drugs* (maternal ingestion), e.g., cytotoxic, *psychosomatic problems* especially stress, severe emotional shock, or emotional instability can influence the viability of the fetus.

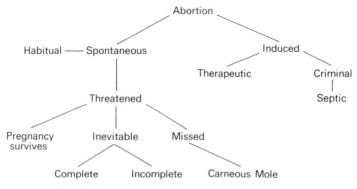

Fig. 12.1. Classification of abortion.

Trauma especially when the uterus is involved or the patient is shocked may lead to abortion. Sometimes coitus causes trauma. An *incompetent* cervix is more common following a previous legal abortion. *Hormonal deficiency* such as a lack of progesterone is probably due to an underdeveloped corpus luteum.

Abortion may be caused by a variety of bacteria or virus. The following organisms are implicated: *Chlamydia trachomatis*, cytomegalovirus, *Toxoplasma gondii*, and *Listeria monocytogenes*.

Deficiencies of copper, zinc and folic acid are also thought to be implicated in abortion, and certainly there is a high incidence of birth defects in women found to have low serum zinc levels.

Threatened abortion

The main symptom of a threatened abortion is that of slight uterine bleeding (Fig. 12.2a). Symptoms of pregnancy are usually present such as amenorrhoea, nausea and breast enlargement. Haemorrhage is usually slight but can be quite heavy and fresh. Pain is not usual but slight pain may be felt.

A vaginal and bimanual examination will be carried out to estimate the degree of dilation of the cervical os. Cervical erosion or a polyp which may be the cause of bleeding will be seen on speculum examination. Pregnancy tests and ultrasound scan will confirm fetal viability. A midstream specimen of urine and a high vaginal swab will be taken so infection can be ruled out as a possible cause.

TREATMENT

The two main principles of treatment are *bedrest* (this reduces mechanical stimuli to the uterus) and mild *sedation*. The patient should be allowed to

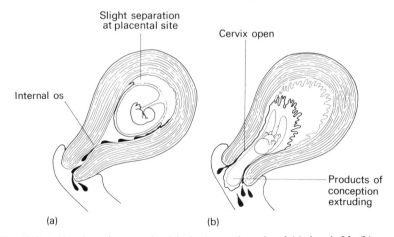

Fig. 12.2. Abortion: threatened, with the internal os closed (a), inevitable (b).

mobilize 48 hours after bleeding has ceased. Any clots or tissue passed by the patient must be saved for inspection. Vulval pads must also be inspected. Enemas and laxatives must *not* be given, as these may intensify the risk of abortion.

The patient may be allowed home after 3-4 days with advice to both the patient and her partner. She should avoid strenuous activity and avoid coitus until after the twelfth week of pregnancy. She should also be advised to contact her doctor if any further bleeding occurs. If bleeding persists and the uterus is contracting painfully then the abortion usually becomes inevitable.

INEVITABLE ABORTION

Abortion becomes inevitable when uterine haemorrhage continues and contractions continue to be strong and painful leading to dilatation of the internal cervical os. Nothing now will prevent abortion occurring. The products of conception which may include fetus, placenta and membranes are extruded from the uterus (Fig. 12.2b). If they are completely extruded this is termed a *complete abortion*. The uterus is now empty and no further treatment is necessary. If the contents are only partially extruded, this is an *incomplete abortion*. In incomplete abortion haemorrhage may be severe, even if this is not the case the patient may become shocked as products of conception distend the cervical canal. The 'Flying Squad' may even be called to hasten the patient's admission to hospital.

Management

The management of a patient suffering from an inevitable abortion will involve:
1 Intravenous replacement of fluid and blood and treatment of shock.
2 Observations of vital signs—temperature, pulse, blood pressure and respirations.
3 Administration of prescribed analgesia and drugs to control uterine haemorrhage—IV/IM ergometrine maleate 0.5 mg or IM ergometrine 500 μg with oxytocin 5 units (Syntometrine).
4 Observation of vaginal bleeding and all tissue passed is vital. Any products of conception in the cervical canal may be removed by the doctor digitally or by sponge-holding forceps at vaginal examination.
5 Withholding food and fluids as the patient will probably have her uterus evacuated under general anaesthesia.
6 Continuous reassurance and support *must* be given.

Blood will be taken for grouping and cross-matching, prior to the patient going to theatre.

Vulval toilet must be performed if necessary.

The patient may be discharged after 24 to 48 hours providing her haemoglobin level is satisfactory. Antibiotics may be prescribed, as sepsis may follow any abortion.

The psychological trauma, which abortion causes both the patient and her partner, must not be overlooked during the urgent phase of her treatment. A period of bereavement will be experienced by a couple looking forward to the birth of their baby and much reassurance will be needed regarding future pregnancies.

MISSED ABORTION

When the embryo or fetus has died in the uterus but the uterus has failed to expel the products of conception this is known as a missed abortion.

The patient who has previously felt herself to be pregnant no longer experiences the symptoms of pregnancy, i.e., nausea and breast changes. She may have had a bout of vaginal bleeding prior to this. The diagnosis is confirmed by a vaginal examination, an ultrasound scan, a Sonicaid (after 12 weeks) and pregnancy tests. On examination the uterus will be found to be smaller than expected for gestational dates. Pregnancy tests are usually negative. Scans will show a defective gestational sac and absence of fetal growth. No fetal heart movement will be seen on ultrasound scan and no fetal heart will be heard via the Sonicaid.

Sometimes the products of conception mass together and are surrounded by old clotted blood; this is referred to as a *carneous mole*, and is an example of a missed abortion.

Management

The situation must be fully explained to the patient who will undoubtedly feel distressed by the thoughts of her baby having died inside her. Three possible lines of treatment exist:

1   Await spontaneous abortion (within 3-4 weeks of the death of the fetus).
2   Stimulate uterine contractions so that abortion takes place.
3   Evacuate the uterus surgically.

If spontaneous abortion is awaited there is a slight risk of hypofibrinogenaemia and intravenous fibrinogen will have to be given to correct the deficiency.

The patient herself is unlikely to want to await spontaneous abortion and will probably opt for an early removal of uterine contents. Surgical evacuation of the uterus may be carried out if this was an early pregnancy, but most gynaecologists prefer to delay a little if possible as surgery can be hazardous. If the pregnancy had progressed to beyond 12-14 weeks uterine contraction may be stimulated by slow intravenous infusion of oxytocin (Syntocinon) or Prostaglandin E_2 (Prostin E_2. These abortifacient drugs will eventually cause the uterus to contract strongly so that all contents are expelled. Side effects from these drugs are usually related to dosage; they include nausea, vomiting and also more severe side effects of uterine rupture and water retention. Whilst the patient is receiving this treatment her vital signs must be observed and the frequency and strength of uterine contractions and vaginal bleeding closely monitored.

Habitual abortion

Abortion is considered habitual or recurrent after 3 or more consecutive pregnancies have terminated in spontaneous abortion, although most patients request attention after 2 abortions. The causes are varied, many of these have been mentioned previously and include uterine abnormalities, incompetent cervix, general maternal illness and hormonal deficiency.

CERVICAL INCOMPETENCE

The cervical canal is found to be dilated and abortion usually occurs in the second trimester around the twentieth week of pregnancy. This is due to incompetence of the cervix.

A procedure may be carried out under general anaesthesia in which a non-absorbable suture encircles the cervix so that the cervical canal remains closed throughout the pregnancy (Shirodkar's suture). This suture can be removed in theatre around the thirty-eighth week allowing normal labour to commence.

There is a slight risk of precipitating irritability of the uterine muscle after this surgical procedure and for this reason a 'uterine sedative' may be prescribed such as ritodrine (Yutopar) or salbutamol (Ventolin). If, however, uterine contractions become severe after insertion of the suture and abortion becomes inevitable it must be removed.

HORMONAL DEFICIENCY

Some authorities believe that recurrent abortion may be caused by deficiency of progesterone for this reason oral progesterone such as dydrogesterone (Duphaston) may be tried, if progesterone deficiency is proven. This treatment though is losing favour with drug safety committees.

Other authorities believe that with adequate rest and diet, and advice on avoiding coitus in the early months the pregnancy will continue. An important aspect of treatment is the restoration of the patient's confidence which will undoubtedly be undermined by previous miscarriages. She may be reassured by the fact that the chances of the pregnancy succeeding are set at 70-80%.

INDUCED ABORTION

Therapeutic abortion

The termination of a pregnancy to safeguard the life of the mother has been held to be legal in Great Britain since 1968 if it was performed by a registered medical practitioner on registered premises. Termination of pregnancy is now legal in many countries, e.g., USA, Australia, Japan and Scandinavia under certain circumstances. In Great Britain the Abortion Act of 1967 permits termination of pregnancy under specific conditions in which the continuance of pregnancy would involve risk to:

1 The life of the pregnant woman.
2 The physical or mental health of the woman.
3 The physical or mental health of the woman's existing children.
4 That there is a substantial risk that the child will be born with physical or mental abnormalities.

Two medical practitioners must certify in good faith that one or more of the above criteria exist before a termination can be performed.

TECHNIQUES

In the first trimester (up to 12 weeks) vacuum aspiration and suction curettage can be used to terminate a pregnancy. In the second trimester it should be noted that the more advanced the gestation the greater the risk to the patient if the pregnancy is terminated. Several techniques are available including intra-amniotic injections, extraamniotic prostaglandins, abdominal hysterotomy and intravenous induction.

Vacuum aspiration

Before the eighth week minimal cervical dilatation is required and the products of conception can easily be aspirated. A local paracervical anaesthetic can be given for this procedure. A metal or plastic (Karman) aspirator is introduced through the cervix and a negative pressure of 0.4-0.6 kg/cm^2 applied. This procedure can be done on an outpatient basis.

Suction curettage

After the eighth week cervical dilation is necessary so that a larger suction curette may be passed into the uterus. A general anaesthetic is needed for this procedure so the patient must be admitted to hospital.

Intraamniotic injections

After first aspirating 200 ml of amniotic fluid, 200 ml of hypertonic saline is injected into the amniotic cavity via the abdomen. This will cause fetal death and abortion usually occurs within 24 hours. This method has considerable dangers such as convulsions from sodium intoxication and cerebral infarction should the saline solution enter the maternal vascular system.

Prostaglandins and urea may also be injected into the amniotic cavity. The procedure is the same as before and in both cases a local anaesthetic such as lignocaine 1 % may be injected into the abdominal tissues prior to intraamniotic injection to reduce discomfort.

Extraamniotic prostaglandins

Prostaglandin E_2 (Prostin E_2) may be introduced into the extraamniotic space via a catheter passed through the cervical os into the uterus. Continuous or intermittent administration (via a Palmer pump) may be effective in causing abortion. Recently prostaglandins in gel introduced into the extraamniotic space has been found to be effective if given 6-hourly until abortion. These methods may be used for termination carried out after 14 weeks.

Administration of prostaglandins may cause nausea, vomiting and diarrhoea. The patient must be admitted to hospital for this procedure as she needs very careful monitoring throughout. It is essential, as in the treatment of missed abortion with oxytocin (Syntocinon) infusion, to monitor uterine contractions as uterine rupture is again a risk.

NB The Palmer pump is a digital syringe pump.

Abdominal hysterotomy

If other methods have failed or if the upper limits for termination (20 weeks) have been reached an abdominal hysterotomy may be chosen. It resembles a caesarean section and carries the same risks as a laparotomy. A hysterotomy leaves a scar on the uterus. The woman is often sterilized at the same time or a pregnant hysterectomy may occasionally be performed.

Intravenous induction

The use of intravenous infusions containing either oxytocin (Syntocinon) or prostaglandins (Prostin E_2) has been mentioned previously in the section on missed abortion.

RISKS

Risks of induced abortion include:
1 Haemorrhage.
2 Cervical damage.
3 Sepsis (especially in criminal abortion).
4 Infertility.
5 Psychological trauma.

CONSCIENTIOUS OBJECTION

The conscientious objection to participation in treatment is a clause in the Great Britain Abortion Act of 1967 which says that no person is obliged to participate in the termination of a pregnancy if they hold a conscientious objection to such a procedure. This clause however makes it clear that a nurse must participate in treatment which is necessary to save the life or prevent grave permanent injury to the physical or mental health of the pregnant woman.

At delivery, spontaneous abortion and termination of pregnancy there is a small amount of fetomaternal bleeding, that is, a transplacental bleed. This results in fetal erythrocytes entering the maternal circulation. If the mother is Rhesus negative and the fetal erythrocytes are Rhesus positive then Rhesus iso-immunization could occur. If so, the mother begins to form antibodies towards these fetal cells. This would mean that haemolytic disease of the newborn would occur in future pregnancies. To prevent this happening 75-100 μg of anti D immunoglobulin is given within 72 hours of delivery or abortion so as to destroy the fetal erythrocytes in the maternal circulation before antibodies can be formed.

Criminal and septic abortion

Uterine infection can occur during *any* stage of abortion but sepsis is much more likely in illegally induced or 'backstreet' abortions. During abortion the natural resistance of the genital tract to infection is impaired and the dangers of a septic abortion are clearly increased if the procedure is carried out without proper regard for *asepsis.*

The risk of infection is further heightened if during the procedure the uterus is incompletely emptied and fragments of tissue are retained. This will cause infection and haemorrhage.

In self-induced abortion the peritoneal cavity may be accidentally entered through the posterior fornix with implements such as knitting needles. Other adjacent structures may also be traumatized. Haemorrhage, salpingitis, peritonitis and septicaemia may all result from criminal interference.

The patient usually gives a history suggestive of an incomplete abortion. Pyrexia and tachycardia may be present. Abdominal tenderness makes vaginal examination painful. Often a purulent offensive vaginal discharge is obvious and the person may look flushed and toxic.

Sepsis may follow any abortion, especially criminal abortion. Further serious complications of septic abortion are bacteraemic (endotoxic shock) caused by organisms such as *E. coli* and exotoxic shock caused by *Clostridium welchii.* For this reason management needs to be active. A high vaginal swab must be taken for culture and sensitivity and antibiotic therapy is commenced. Evacuation of the uterus will be delayed for 24 hours until antibiotics become effective unless there is continued heavy bleeding. This will lessen the risk of infecting organisms entering the blood stream causing endotoxic shock.

If endotoxic shock does occur the patient is best treated in an intensive care unit where blood gases and arterial and central venous pressures (CVP) and urinary function can be monitored. Initially though treatment must be administered where the patient is.

NURSING MANAGEMENT

1 This patient will require bedrest and analgesia may be needed.
2 It is essential to encourage a high fluid intake and record urinary output.
3 Four-hourly observation of temperature and pulse is necessary. Vaginal bleeding must be monitored.
4 Vulval toilet is needed because of the offensive vaginal discharge.
5 All necessary nursing care, including oral hygiene and care of pressure areas.

Septic abortion unfortunately may result in chronic pelvic sepsis or pelvic inflammatory disease (PID), and many women may remain debilitated for several months afterwards. Infertility may be a problem.

Nursing care

A patient undergoing termination of pregnancy needs particular nursing care following routine admission procedures. The method chosen for the termination, in this case, is an extraamniotic instillation of prostaglandin (Prostin E_2) following prior ripening of the cervix with prostaglandin pessaries.

PREPARATION OF THE PATIENT

Psychological

The psychological preparation of the patient is of paramount importance as inevitably considerable guilt is attached to the decision to terminate a pregnancy. Many prejudices exist in society towards abortion. Religious and ethical concepts may create considerable conflict and pressure for the woman. Recent publicity may lead many women to believe that it will become increasingly more difficult to obtain an abortion in the future.

When a woman comes into hospital for termination of pregnancy she may be in a state of emotional stress, this may not always be apparent in her behaviour, but the nurse must be aware that stress exists. Time must be spent reassuring the patient and answering her questions.

Physical

The physical preparation of the patient involves the following procedures:
1 Vulval and perineal shave may be done followed by a bath.
2 Bisacodyl suppositories or phosphate enema to evacuate the bowel.
3 Dress patient in theatre gown.
4 Encourage voiding of urine prior to the termination process.

5 Prostaglandin (dinoprostone 3 mg) pessaries per vaginam if prescribed. (As these pessaries facilitate abortion administration is the responsibility of the medical staff.)

The patient will lie in the dorsal position with one pillow, knees flexed and thighs abducted. Sterile towels are draped over the thighs and lower abdomen. A Cusco's bilvalve speculum is passed and a good light is provided so that the cervix can be visualized.
Then:
1 A Foley catheter 12-14 FG is passed into the uterine cavity via the external os. The balloon is inflated accordingly.
2 Next the distal end of the Foley catheter is connected to a length of sterile nylon tubing, which in turn is connected to a syringe primed with prostaglandin solution (Prostin E_2).
3 The syringe is placed in position on a syringe pump which is preset to deliver a measured amount over a period of time. These procedures are the responsibility of a medical practitioner. Settings may vary and the following is one example: 1-2 ml prostaglandin/hour for 6 hours then 2-2.5 ml prostaglandin/hour until abortion.

The patient may be settled comfortably whilst she awaits abortion. This is obviously a very trying time for her but her anxiety will be lessened if she is prepared for the sequence of events which will follow. She will require a great deal of support from nursing staff throughout this procedure. Suggestions on how the waiting time can be passed as pleasantly as possible will be appreciated by the patient. She may also appreciate her partner being with her for some of the time. Fluids and light diet may be given at this early stage as abortion can take between 12 to 18 hours. The patient should be allowed to sleep inbetween observation procedures during the night.

Hourly observations will include recording:
1 Blood pressure and pulse.
2 Vaginal bleeding.
3 Uterine contractions.

Other observations include urinary output (a full bladder will cause discomfort and inhibit abortion,) the degree of nausea or vomiting and pain. Antimetics are frequently needed during administration of prostaglandins. Analgesia will be prescribed (Pethedine is the drug of choice) as uterine contractions become stronger.

Infection is a possible side effect of termination of pregnancy, a pyrexia will be detected by 4-hourly observation of temperature. The risk of infection is minimized by maintaining vulval hygiene, the patient will benefit from frequent vulval toilet and the application of a sterile vulval pad once vaginal bleeding has commenced.

When strong uterine contractions are established the Foley catheter may be extruded from the cervix and the membranes ruptured. Passage of the fetus and placenta should follow but often the placenta is retained in the uterus. Adequate analgesia must be given as required. At this point blood loss must be carefully estimated. Fluids will now be witheld if abortion is incomplete and surgical evacuation of the uterus is necessary. Syntometrine 1 ml IM may be prescribed to control any bleeding, the patient is then prepared for theatre in the usual way.

Any tissue passed by the patient will be saved and inspected for completeness.

DELIVERY OF A NONVIABLE FETUS

A qualified nurse should be with the patient during the delivery of a nonviable fetus, and the doctor on call notified. *Strict* asepsis must be maintained throughout the procedure.

Equipment

The following equipment will be required.
Sterile pack containing:
2 large towels
Cotton wool swabs
Container for antiseptic lotion
Receiver
2 pairs artery forceps
1 pair scissors
1 Cusco's speculum
1 sponge-holding forceps
1 pair sterile gloves
Antiseptic lotion—Chlorhexidine 5 % in dilution at 38°C
Jar for specimen with histopathology card

Method

For the delivery of a nonviable fetus:
1 Position the patient: dorsal with one pillow, covering the upper half of the patient's body.
2 Ask patient to flex her knees and abduct her thighs.
3 Drape the area with sterile towels.
4 Allow the fetus to be delivered, usually spontaneously into a receiver.
5 Allow a short time for the placenta to separate and be expelled.
6 If the placenta has not yet been expelled clamp the umbilical cord with artery forceps/clamps and cut in between the two. Do **not** attempt to pull on the umbilical cord, allow natural expulsion of the placenta.

7 Swab the vulval and perineal areas with antiseptic lotion—provide a sterile vulval pad.

8 Check the patient's blood pressure and pulse.

9 Leave the patient warm and settled and allow her to rest, after comforting her.

If a doctor is in attendance during the delivery he or she may attempt to remove the placenta manually or pass a Cusco's speculum and remove the placenta with the sponge-holding forceps, once separation occurs. If the placenta has been retained the patient must be prepared for surgical evacuation of the uterus.

The fetus must be placed in a jar and dispatched to the laboratory with the completed histopathology card as soon as possible.

HYDATIDIFORM MOLE

A hydatidiform mole occurs when, for some unexplained reason, a normal pregnancy is replaced by a mole-like formation, of a mass of multiple small vessicles resembling grapes which fill the uterus (Fig. 12.3). These small vessicles (Fig. 12.4) which are proliferations of chorionic villi are full of fluid and nutrients which, had the pregnancy continued normally, would have nourished the fetus, via the placenta. In a hydatidiform mole no fetus can be seen on ultrasonography and the uterus appears larger than dates suggest.

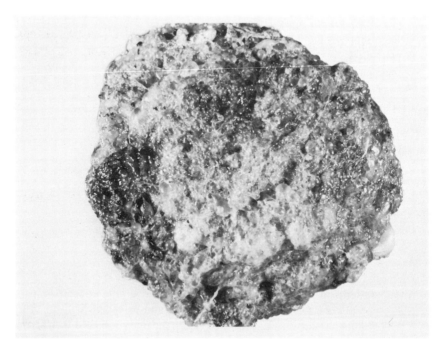

Fig. 12.3. A hydatidiform mole.

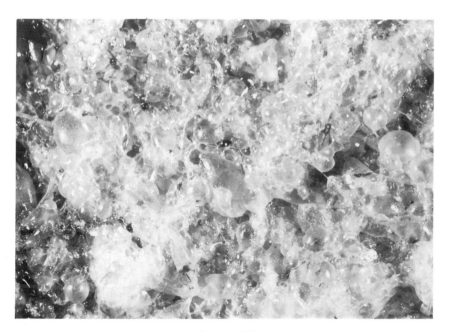

Fig. 12.4. Close-up of the vesicles of a hydatidiform mole.

Incidence

In the United Kingdom, a hydatidiform mole occurs in approximately 1 in 2000 pregnancies. The incidence is far greater in Far Eastern countries and the Philippines.

Clinical features

A patient with a hydatidiform mole may present with:
1 Normal signs and symptoms of pregnancy.
2 Nausea and vomiting which may be exaggerated.
3 Intermittent vaginal bleeding.
4 Passage of ruptured vessicles. This is rare but all matter passed per vaginam must be carefully examined.

Diagnosis

Diagnosis is confirmed by:
1 Ultrasonography—no fetal heart heard, no fetal parts seen.
2 Pregnancy strongly positive even in × 100 dilution.
3 Uterus is rather bigger than dates suggest and on palpation feels 'boggy'.
   Haemorrhage may be profuse because of the invasive action of the trophoblastic tissue.

Treatment

Once the diagnosis is confirmed the mole must be removed as soon as possible, occasionally spontaneous abortion may take place but in all cases surgical evacuation to ensure complete emptying of the uterus is necessary. However the uterus is emptied, bleeding may be profuse and blood transfusion is often required.

In women over 40 years of age a hysterectomy is usually performed.

Follow-up

The greatest danger of a hydatidiform mole is the tendency for it to undergo malignant change and become a chorion epithelioma. This is thought to occur in 5-10 % of cases. The patient must therefore be followed up for at least 2 years after diagnosis.

For the first 6 months the patient should have her urine tested for human chorionic-gonadotrophin (HCG)—the presence of which would confirm continuing trophoblastic activity and possibly malignant change. Follow-up of the patient will be arranged on the basis of the results of the urinary tests, or a return of her symptoms. More usually the level of urinary HCG returns to normal within 2-6 months.

During the follow-up period the patient must be urged not to become pregnant as this would seriously confuse the picture should a positive pregnancy test result.

13 Sexual Problems

As with all sexual problems an organic cause must first be excluded even though the difficulty may be psychosomatic in origin. The problems considered in this chapter are dyspareunia, apareunia, vaginismus, frigidity, and rape.

DYSPAREUNIA

Dyspareunia may be defined as painful or difficult sexual intercourse. It may be superficial or deep. This may be caused by:

1 Vulval or vaginal conditions such as vulvitis or a vaginitis caused by monilial or trichomonal infections.

2 Urethral conditions such as urethritis, urethral caruncle or urethral prolapse.

3 Postmenopausal atrophy or blockage of the Bartholin's glands or ducts.

4 Anatomical narrowing of the introitus. This may be due to a rigid hymenal ring or scarring of the perineum following episiotomy or perineorrhaphy.

Superficial dyspareunia

Superficial (introital) dyspareunia, that is, pain on first intercourse may simply be due to a lack of lubrication and is easily remedied by the use of a lubricant such as water soluble jelly. Lubrication may also be helpful if dryness is due to postmenopausal atrophy.

TREATMENT

All patients who seek advice on sexual matters need tactful and sympathetic handling, it may have taken months or even years for a woman to pluck up enough courage to consult her doctor about her problem.

If reassurance is given throughout the patient may be able to relax so that a gentle vulval and vaginal examination can be carried out, but occasionally digital examination is impossible. At this point any anatomical introital narrowing will be obvious. Surgical treatment (Fenton's operation) will be successful in widening the introitus.

If no obvious organic cause is found further time must be spent with the patient trying to discover a cause and at the same time building up her confidence. Often a seemingly tight introitus, which often follows an episiotomy is successfully treated by vaginal dilation. The dilators are made of plastic (Fig. 13.1) or glass (Fig. 13.2) and are graduated in size. The patient is taught how to lubricate and insert the dilators starting with the smallest size eventually working towards the largest.

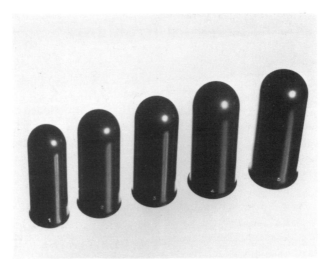

Fig. 13.1. Vaginal dilators made of plastic and graduated.

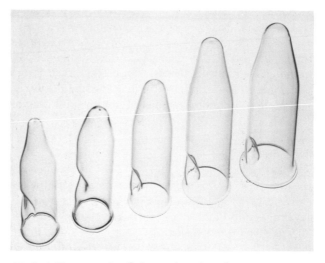

Fig. 13.2. Vaginal dilators made of glass and graduated.

Deep dyspareunia

With deep dyspareunia pain is felt when the erect penis is inserted fully into the vagina. Possible causes are as follows:

1 Pelvic inflammatory disease (PID).
2 Endometriosis.
3 Pelvic tumours.

4 Retroverted uterus with prolapsed ovaries (into the pouch of Douglas).

5 Scar tissue from radiotherapy or previous vaginal surgery.

Treatment of deep dyspareunia is of the underlying cause and this is dealt with under the relevant sections.

APAREUNIA

Apareunia is in itself a symptom which implies that normal coitus cannot be performed. This is because there is either an organic obstruction or a psychological inhibition. This psychological inhibition usually manifests itself as vaginismus. This is a severe spasm of the levator ani in the area surrounding the lower vagina. In extreme cases such is the intensity of muscular spasm that tight adduction of the legs occurs. These pains are so profoundly distressing that the response at future attempts is made more and more difficult. The woman's confidence in her own sexual ability is gradually eroded as each attempt ends in failure.

Often the cause is sheer ignorance of sexual behaviour, clumsy attempts at first coitus or more seriously, an unfortunate experience in the past such as sexual assault or rape. The patient and her husband must both be made aware of the exact nature of their problem. It may be advisable for husband and wife to be seen separately at first so that they might freely reveal any feelings of guilt, fear, ignorance or anxiety. Eventually the couple should be seen together so that each is fully aware of the other's feelings, and both benefit together from sex education. Psychosexual counselling is a skill which requires a sound knowledge of normal sexuality as well as a knowledge of specific sexual problems. Although nurses will not be expected to be psychosexual counsellors in the strictest sense, they should be able to identify sexual problems and be active in helping to correct any mistaken views on sexuality. Many patients will expect nurses to be able to answer their questions.

During investigation and treatment it is wise to forbid any further attempts at intercourse since further frustration may hinder therapy. In this period of abstinence the woman may be taught how to use vaginal dilators, but she must be regularly supervized so that progress can be assessed.

FRIGIDITY

Frigidity may sometimes be confused with dyspareunia but essentially it is an absence of libido or sexual arousal. Libido may be affected by many circumstances, i.e., intense worry about family matters, fatigue or environmental factors. General health also affects libido but by far the commonest cause is one of psychological origin.

Treatment must be based on thorough investigation; a psychiatrist may be involved if a psychiatric problem is discovered, and again a skilled psychosexual counsellor may be needed to spend time with both partners discovering their sexual attitudes and resolving any conflict which might exist between them. All

nurses should be able to explain to the patient that after gynaecological operations libido may be temporarily decreased but that all that is needed is a short
period of adjustment, usually 6 weeks is sufficient.

RAPE

Rape is an expression of physical violence, not sexual desire. In rape a man can
of course achieve sexual gratification but the woman has been used merely as a
passive object from which sexual satisfaction has been obtained. This act of
violence has a tremendous impact upon the victim's physical and psychological
states and far reaching effects upon her family. A rape victim may even be
stigmatized by her close relatives and society because the nature of rape is so very
difficult for those directly involved to come to terms with.

A definition of rape might be useful here as a perspective as various definitions
exist. I quote a few which exist: 'the unlawful sexual intercourse of a woman
without her consent, by force, fear or fraud.' (Butterworth's Medical Dictionary). 'Forcible or fraudulent sexual intercourse especially imposed on
women.' (The Concise Oxford Dictionary).

The law

In the United States of America, the term statutory rape exists, that is, sexual
intercourse with a girl below the age of consent. In the United Kingdom sexual
intercourse or attempted sexual intercourse of a girl under 13 years is unlawful,
also of a girl between 13 and 16 years. The latter may be open to argument if the
accused claims he had reason to believe the girl to be over 16 years, provided,
that he himself is under the age of 23 years at that time and had not previously
been charged with a similar offence.

Other important points of law are that no force is needed for rape to have taken
place in females who are under 13 years, or females who are mentally subnormal.
Neither has full penetration or ejaculation to take place, mere entry to the vulva
is sufficient.

Recently some legal minds have thought that offenders should be charged
simply with physical assault so that spurious arguments on what constitutes rape
such as whether the woman was sleeping, intoxicated or dressed or behaving in a
provocative fashion, are avoided.

There are thought to be up to 10 times more cases of rape occur than the actual
number reported. The reasons for this are complex but unsympathetic attitudes
of police and hospital personnel and possibly family members may be partly to
blame. A woman will quite understandably shrink from further humiliation
which close investigation will bring. She may be forced to seek professional help
if because of rough coitus vaginal and perineal tears have resulted. Despite all the
physical and psychological trauma suffered by the victim she may still be met
with hostility from those she needs most at such a time.

Examination

Examination should take place as soon as possible after the incident. She must give her consent and be examined in the presence of a third party. After the woman has been allowed to give her own account of the incidence the following detailed examination will take place:

1 State of clothing.
2 Emotional state.
3 Evidence of bruises.
4 State of finger nails.
5 Vulval condition.
6 Microscopic evidence of semen.
7 Microscopic evidence of sexually transmitted disease.
8 Specimens of hair and pubic hair.

The sequence of legal events which takes place once rape has been proven is not relevant here. A nurse would be concerned with this woman's physical and mental well-being from this point onwards, and should be aware that in many of Great Britain's major cities rape crisis centres exist which may provide emotional support and legal advice for rape victims.

14 Fertility and Family Planning

INFERTILITY

It has been estimated that approximately 10 % of marriages are childless, that is, one or other of the partners appear to be infertile. If a woman has never been able to conceive, her infertility is said to be *primary*. If conception has taken place, whatever the outcome, and then infertility follows this is said to be *secondary* infertility.

Recent scientific advances have helped solve many problems of infertility so that many couples can now be helped. It is considered reasonable to commence investigations into infertility if conception has not occurred after 12-18 months despite regular coitus without contraceptives. It is important to remember that fertility reaches its peak between the ages of 20-25, therefore if a couple in their 30s seek advice about infertility investigation becomes more urgent.

Infertility can create great stress and anxiety within a partnership. Prolonged and intensive investigation may occasionally prove too much for the stability of the partnership. There is a tendency now to adopt simple schemes of investigation and uncomplicated treatment regimes. It is vital that 'blame' is not apportioned to either the husband or wife whatever the outcome of investigation. Peter Speck in *Loss and Grief in Medicine* says that some couples may show a marked reaction to the fact that they are unable to conceive. This point should be borne in mind when dealing with the infertile couple.

Causes of male infertility

LACK OF VIABLE SPERMATAZOA

Spermatogenesis can be affected by many different factors, overwork, smoking or excessive alcohol consumption may result in a low sperm count, *oligospermia*. Scrotal temperature also affects spermatogenesis because testicular function is impaired by high temperatures. *Azoospermia*, absence of sperm, may be caused by undescended testes, chromosomal hypothalamic or pituitary disorders. Seminal analysis should be carried out before further investigation is instigated (Table 14.1). A fresh specimen should be obtained by masturbation, after abstaining from coitus for at least 3-4 days. The specimen must be ejaculated into a clean glass jar, kept at body temperature and dispatched to the laboratory within 2 hours.

FAILURE OF INSEMINATION

The cause of infertility may be one of faulty insemination and not one of faulty spermatogenesis. Failure of insemination occurs in conditions such as: impo-

Table 14.1 Semen analysis

Evaluation	Normal value
Volume	3-7 ml
pH	7.4-7.8
Sperm count	60,000,000-200,000,000 ml
Motility	50 % active motility after 5 hours
Form	90 % normal formation

tence, premature ejaculation, hypospadias, and obstruction of the male genital tract. Retrograde ejaculation (into the bladder) of seminal fluid may occur after prostatectomy.

TREATMENT

Any obvious underlying cause must be treated. Advice on life style and social habits may be very effective, wearing of loose cotton underpants and avoidance of hot baths may be simply all that is needed in men with low sperm counts. In men with azoospermia artificial insemination by a donor (AID) may be suggested to the couple as an alternative to adoption.

Causes of female infertility

A pregnancy requires that an ovum of good quality be fertilized by a healthy sperm. The act of ova and sperm uniting is called conception. From this point onwards there must be an unobstructed passage along the uterine tube, so that the zygote, now so called, can journey to the uterus to implant and obtain its basic nourishment through the chorionic villi. Ovarian function is vital in preparing the endometrium and uterine environment to receive the by now developing embryo. Pituitary and hypothalamic disorders will inevitably affect ovarian function and must be considered when investigating infertility (Fig. 14.1).

ANXIETY

When a couple is trying to conceive their anxiety is often increased if each month brings disappointment instead of joy. This anxiety is often further increased by friends and relatives repeatedly enquiring about their childlessness. Anxiety affects libido, diminished libido increases anxiety and tension thus a vicious circle is set up. The reason for most couples success shortly after adopting a baby is that tubal spasm is relieved once anxiety is lessened, tubal spasm having caused the initial infertility: 'Tense patient, tense tubes.'

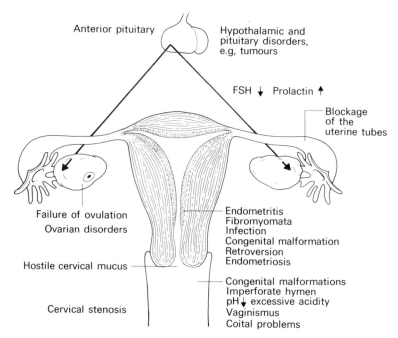

Fig. 14.1. Causes of female infertility.

IMMUNOLOGICAL FACTORS

Immunological factors may operate at any stage of the human reproductive process. Gametes, the fertilized ovum and hormones are all antigens which might stimulate antibody formation in the woman. Antibody formation may lead to destruction of the sperm. Normally physiological mechanisms operate to overcome this immune response, but if these mechanisms fail, infertility results.

COITAL TECHNIQUES

When coitus always takes place at times other than ovulation, conception is unlikely to occur. Ignorance of coital techniques may result in faulty insemination; some women seeking advice on account of infertility are found not to have consummated their marriage.

Investigations

CLINICAL EXAMINATION

A clinical examination will be carried out and will include:
Exclusion of pelvic abnormalities
Cervical cytology

Assessment of general health
Assessment of nutritional state

DETAILED HISTORY

A history will be taken from the couple which will detail:
Coital behaviour
Sexual attitudes
Previous contraception
Social history

BASAL BODY TEMPERATURE

Before exhaustive tests are embarked upon a simple test to establish whether ovulation is taking place may be done. The patient is asked to take her temperature, on waking, each morning starting on the first day of her period. If she records her temperature on a chart for three successive cycles a pattern should emerge. If she is ovulating there should be a noticeable drop in temperature at around day 14 followed by an immediate rise of approximately 0.5°C which is usually sustained until her next period; this is evidence of corpus luteum formation. Basal body temperature is an inexpensive index of ovulation.

CERVICAL MUCUS TESTS

A sample of cervical mucus may be taken and placed on a glass slide. Due to the action of oestrogens this mucus crystallizes when it dries and forms a pattern which is called *ferning*. Progesterone prevents the formation of this pattern so that if ferning appears in the second half of the cycle anovulation is suspected. Ferning therefore should only be seen around ovulation time.

VAGINAL SMEAR

Distinct cellular changes can be demonstrated if ovulation has taken place. These changes are brought about by hormonal activity. Papanicolaou's staining method is used.

BLOOD TESTS

Estimations of blood levels of gonadatrophic hormones, follicle stimulating hormone (FSH) and luteinizing hormone (LH), are indicators of pituitary and hypothalamic function. If hypothalamic function fails FSH and LH levels fall and because the normal hypothalamus inhibits prolactin secretion a serum prolactin assay will show an abnormal increase. Another test that will confirm ovulation is an estimation of serum progesterone, after the fourteenth day of a 28-day cycle.

ENDOMETRIAL BIOPSY (PREMENSTRUAL)

A small fragment of the endometrium can be obtained by using a small biopsy curette, the Vabra aspirator. If the fragment proves to be secretory endometrium this establishes that ovulation is taking place. The procedure can be done on an outpatient basis. The biopsied specimens should also be cultured for tuberculosis. A dilatation and curettage (D & C) will serve the same purpose, if performed in the second half of the cycle.

LAPAROSCOPY

Direct visualization of the contents of the pelvis will reveal any abnormality which may affect fertility, such as adhesions occluding the fimbriae or endometriosis. Likewise, tubal patency can also be demonstrated during laparoscopy. See also pp. 207–8.

TUBAL PATENCY TESTS

An informative tubal patency test is the hysterosalpingogram, once genital tuberculosis has been excluded. Radio opaque dye is introduced into the uterus via a cervical cannula. An X-ray screen or films taken at intervals will demonstrate the outline of the uterine cavity and uterine tubes then show spillage of the dye from both tubes, if there is no blockage. Tubal insufflation with CO_2 (Rubin's test) is less widely used these days as there is no indication with this test of the *site* of the obstruction in the case of a blockage.

POSTCOITAL TESTS

At ovulation cervical mucus should be clear and increased in amount, less viscid, more alkaline and in general receptive to sperm. A microscopic examination of postcoital cervical mucus (Huhner test) will confirm whether or not the sperms are surviving in the cervical environment. This test must be done at ovulation and within 2 hours of coitus. It may be found that there are sperm antibodies in cervical mucus.

In vitro postcoital tests can be performed. On the calculated day of ovulation a specimen of mucus is mixed with fresh sperm on a glass slide. Sperm activity and their ability to invade the mucus is observed through a microscope. If it is noted that the sperm die as soon as they contact the mucus this will be the cause of infertility.

Treatment

The treatment of infertility depends upon the outcome of investigation. Organic diseases such as fibromyomata or endometriosis will be treated appropriately. Pelvic infections will be treated with antibiotics.

INDUCTION OF OVULATION

If a woman is found to be anovulatory treatment is directed towards induction of ovulation. The choice of drug will depend upon the cause of the ovulatory failure. If the cause is a low level of FSH, clomiphene citrate (Clomid) a synthetic preparation may produce an increase in FSH production and thus induce ovulation. Menotrophin (Pergonal), a preparation of human gonadotrophin, may be also given. Throughout treatment biochemical monitoring is essentially carried out by measurement of either urinary or plasma hormone levels. Monitoring of treatment will confirm that ovulation has been induced and also avoid hyperstimulation which could occur resulting in multiple pregnancies.

Another drug which may be prescribed is bromocriptine. This is indicated when the serum prolactin level is abnormally high. Bromocriptine is capable of restoring normal menstruation and fertility.

BLOCKAGE OF UTERINE TUBES

If the cause of infertility is blockage of the uterine tubes it may be possible to clear this by tubal insufflation. If not, tubal surgery may be necessary and may take the form of:

Salpingolysis for separation of adhesions around the tube.
Salpingostomy for creation of a new opening at the distal end of the tube.
Tubal reimplantation for congenital obstruction.
Tubal reanastomosis for reversal of sterilization.

IMPENETRABLE MUCUS

If the cervical mucus is found to be impenetrable to sperm, oestrogen which liquefies viscid mucus may be given in the form of ethinyloestradiol. An excessively acid vaginal environment may be lessened by precoital sodium bicarbonate douches.

NB   One of the newest drugs to be used in the treatment of anovulatory infertility is tamoxifen (Nolvadex).

ARTIFICIAL INSEMINATION

The highly controversial issue of artificial insemination presents many ethical, moral and religious dilemmas. The demand for artificial insemination by a donor (AID) has increased over the years. The reasons for this may be that it is more acceptable to the infertile couple or that fewer babies are available for adoption. It may be that a combination of reasons make AID a more attractive proposition. It is an irony that whereas many couples experience frustration and disappointment because they are childless, the number of pregnancies which are therapeutically terminated each year in this and other countries is staggering.

Artificial insemination by the husband (AIH) may also be performed. This is direct insemination with sperm from the husband which may be undertaken if the wife is ovulating and the husband's sperm is healthy.

By husband

Probable indications for AIH will include:
    Coital difficulties
    Premature ejaculation
    Male impotence
    Hypospadias
    Unexplained poor postcoital tests
    Cervical stenosis
If the husband has to undergo radiotherapy his sperm may be obtained and stored whilst awaiting a suitable time for insemination.

TECHNIQUE

The spermatazoa is collected, usually by masturbation, into a jar. The sperm is then drawn up into a syringe and introduced into the cervical canal or vaginal vault. It is possible for the couple to perform this technique together if normal coitus is difficult due to disability. Insemination may have to be repeated several times before conception takes place. Insemination is best performed on the day closest to ovulation and this is more accurately planned if the basal body temperature is taken, to confirm that ovulation has taken place.

By donor

Artificial insemination by a donor presents many more moral dilemmas. Doctors and nurses may have religious or moral objections and many people may find the whole idea distasteful. It is however a way of bringing happiness and fulfilment to infertile couples. Artificial insemination clinics have now been established in several centres and more are being organized.

Before a couple are considered for AID they must be fully interviewed so that an assessment of their attitudes may be made. Some authorities feel that it is better if the couple suggest donor insemination themselves. It is important for the couple to appreciate that the success rate is approximately 30 %, although it can be much higher. This means that they must be prepared for possible disappointment.

AID is indicated when the woman is normally fertile and the husband sterile. This means that healthy sperm must be donated by a male who is physically fit and of average intelligence. Donor characteristics must also include a normal genetic make-up and a good sperm count. Some clinics match donor characteristics with those of the infertile husband. The donor must, of course, be prepared to cooperate in the AID programme. Donor and recipient should be and remain completely anonymous for all time.

The procedure is the same as AIH. Intracervical insemination is the most usual method. The donor sperm, drawn up into a cannula is deposited in the cervix and vaginal vault, the woman is then allowed to rest for 15 minutes before going home.

As AID continues to provoke much debate, unfortunately emotive language is being used in this connection which can only serve to obscure the real issues. Phrases such as 'donor panels of top sires', or 'superior seed catalogues' (World Medicine 1982) contribute very little that is constructive to the continuing arguments.

IN VITRO FERTILIZATION

Literally *in vitro* means in glass. *In vitro* fertilization therefore means that ova and sperm unite within a test tube under controlled laboratory conditions; hence the term *test tube baby*.

In the United Kingdom Mr Patrick Steptoe and Dr Robert Edwards were both largely responsible for the early advances in *in vitro* fertilization. They began their historic work in the late 1960s but it was not until 1978 that the world's first test tube baby was born at Oldham District General Hospital. In September 1982 a fertility clinic in Cambridge announced the birth of its fiftieth test tube baby. This clinic was set up by Mr Steptoe and Dr Edwards both now regarded internationally as the pioneers of test tube work. In Australia Professor Carl Wood and Dr Allan Trounson have also had remarkable success. Both Australia and the USA are developing and researching into *in vitro* fertilization programmes.

TECHNIQUE

Fertility drugs are often prescribed so that several mature Graafian follicles are ensured for in vitro fertilization. This also ensures that spare follicles are available. At an appropriate time a maturing follicle (ova) is recovered from the ovary via a laparoscope and placed in a test tube.

After a short period of time (approximately 2 hours) at an incubation temperature of 37°C the, by now, fully matured ova is fertilized by the husband's sperm. Semen must be freshly obtained or frozen sperm allowed to thaw. The sperm, between 10,000 and 100,000, are added to the test tube which is again incubated at blood heat. Eventually the spermatazoa may penetrate the ova so that fertilization takes place. From this point the fertilized ova is allowed to divide and subdivide until it becomes a blastocyst and eventually a viable human embryo.

After approximately 40 hours embryo transfer is undertaken. The embryo is deposited high up in the uterine cavity via a fine cervical catheter. If the transfer is successful a normal pregnancy will result. The use of electron microscopy now makes it possible to determine the quality and sex of the embryo prior to reimplantation.

Implications

In vitro fertilization was initially intended solely for women with uterine tube blockage, whatever the cause. Now a wider and very debatable application is envisaged whereby a woman with nonfunctioning ovaries may be helped by this technique provided a suitable oöcyte donor can be found.

Many ethical issues are being raised and concern is being expressed about what the future holds for work of this nature, so much so that a Government enquiry has been set up to investigate these issues. Issues which are causing great concern are the existence of sperm and embryo *banks.* The major ethical questions being asked are, to whom do the frozen spermatazoa and embryos belong? Do embryos have any rights? Another possibility causing concern is that embryos may be allowed to develop to a point where organs are formed enabling research to take place into organic disease. This inevitably results in death of the embryo. The medical profession and many other lay and professional groups are looking for some clear legal and moral guidelines for the future. Many feel that developments have already gone 'beyond the framework of human ethics'.

FAMILY PLANNING

Giving advice to patients on family planning is an essential part of gynaecological nursing. Every second there are two more births than deaths in the world which means that the population increases by approximately 200,000 each day. The world's population continues to double in size, almost increasing by its own momentum. Natural resources are dwindling and the world's food supplies are unequally shared. Family planning is therefore a matter of world-wide concern.

In recent years newly developed methods of contraception have created the need for a professional service which can provide advice on what is essentially a very personal matter. Postgraduate courses are now available which enable doctors and nurses to study and research methods of contraception. Nurses must be knowledgeable not only about methods available but also capable of explaining simply the facts to their clients who will primarily be concerned with the convenience, safety and effectiveness of a given method. A selection of contraceptives available are shown in figure 14.2.

The large number of abortions which are carried out in many countries each year confirms that many married and unmarried women find pregnancy intolerable yet neglect to ensure that they or their partners use an effective method of contraception. In fact abortion is the most widely used contraceptive. When invited to give advice on family planning methods it is important to respect the individual's preference. They should not be coerced into using a method which seems to them unacceptable or morally wrong. Family planning may include advice on abortion, subfertility or psychosexual counselling. These issues have been dealt with in previous chapters.

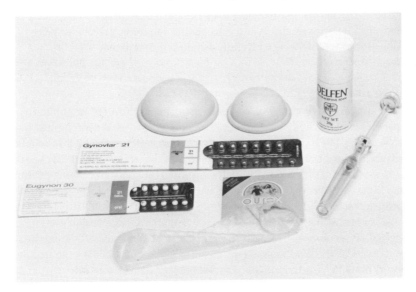

Fig. 14.2. Various methods of contraception which are available.

Principles of contraception

There are three main principles of contraception: prevention of fertilization, prevention of ovulation, and prevention of implantation. The prevention of fertilization requires that ova and sperm do not meet.

Prevention of fertilization

COITUS INTERRUPTUS

Coitus interruptus or the withdrawal method depends upon withdrawal of the penis from the vagina immediately prior to ejaculation. It requires a certain degree of self-discipline and may lead to unsatisfactory sexual intercourse. This method also has a high failure rate as sperm may escape from the penis just before withdrawal or a pregnancy may result if semen is deposited in the vulval area. It is however a popular method requiring no premeditation or appliance.

CONDOM

The condom or sheath can be a very effective method of contraception with the added advantage of affording some protection against sexually transmitted disease. Condoms are usually made of fine latex, which may be lubricated, and are disposable. It is important when advising on the usage of the condom to stress that it must be applied when the penis is fully erect and held in place when withdrawing so that semen does not escape. The effectiveness of the condom is increased if the female partner uses a spermicide. The disadvantages with this method are that spontaneity is lost and genital sensation may be impaired. In addition if the condom is not carefully handled it may burst.

DIAPHRAGM

The diaphragm or Dutch cap is currently enjoying an upsurge in popularity as the problems associated with taking oral contraceptives are becoming more widely known. The diaphragm is attractive in that it allows the woman to retain responsibility for her own protection. To be effective it is essential that the diaphragm is of the correct size and initially it is fitted by a doctor or family planning nurse. Time must be allowed for supervized practice and the user must be able to insert and remove the diaphragm before she leaves the clinic. It is important that she is able to check that her cervix is covered by the diaphragm each time it is inserted. Prior to insertion a layer of spermicidal cream should be applied to both surfaces of the diaphragm. Because it is made of rubber it may perish in time and must be regularly inspected. To prevent deterioration the diaphragm should be washed thoroughly and dried then stored in a specially provided container.

Another similar device which may be used to prevent sperm from entering the cervix is the cervical cap which fits directly onto the cervix. For this reason it is less easy for the user to fit and therefore is much less popular.

SPERMICIDES

With spermicides a chemical barrier is provided which will destroy any sperm deposited in the vagina. Creams, foams, pessaries or foaming tablets may be inserted into the vagina approximately 5 minutes before intercourse so that time is allowed for them to melt. In general spermicides are much more effective when used in conjunction with other methods of contraception such as the condom or the diaphragm.

Recent developments in barrier protection include a contraceptive sponge impregnated with a spermicidal agent and secondly a square of material impregnated with spermicide (C-film). The sponge is undergoing trials to evaluate its safety and effectiveness. C-film which is applied to the tip of the penis or over the cervical os is considered ineffective and is not recommended.

RHYTHM (OVULATION OR SAFE PERIOD)

The rhythm or safe period method is attractive to couples who prefer not to use any mechanical aids or to take the contraceptive pill. It does however rely upon a knowledge of biology and a basic understanding of the ovulatory cycle. The aim is to restrict intercourse to the infertile days of the menstrual cycle, that is, to prohibit intercourse at the time of ovulation. It is essential therefore to predict the time of ovulation, this may be done by the calendar method, the temperature method or testing the cervical mucus.

Calendar method

The calendar method involves calculating the menstrual cycle for a period of 6-12 months. The precise length of each cycle is carefully recorded, counting the first day of bleeding as day 1. The high risk time begins 18 days *back* from the end of the *shortest* cycle and 11 days from the end of the *longest*. If the shortest cycle is 25 days (25 − 18 = 7) and the longest cycle is 31 days (31 − 11 = 20), day 7 becomes the first unsafe day and day 20 becomes the last unsafe day.

The greatest drawback of this method is that it depends upon the cycle staying within the calculated cycle pattern.

Temperature method

The temperature is taken each day, before rising. A cup of tea or cigarette must not be taken before doing this. A special fertility thermometer may be used and the reading recorded on a temperature chart (Fig. 14.3).

Ovulation is confirmed by a rise in temperature of 0.5°C which persists for several days. Coitus is unsafe before and for at least 3 days after ovulation. This method is considered more reliable than the calendar method but allows fewer safe days.

Cervical mucus (Billings method)

Alterations in the quality of cervical mucus correlates closely with ovulation. Cervical mucus is scanty and sticky for most of the cycle but immediately prior to ovulation and for a few days afterwards it becomes slippery and more profuse. This is called ovulation mucus. This method depends upon an understanding of this principle and a daily self-examination of the cervical mucus. It is a method which is still on trial and which is presently being evaluated by the International Planned Parenthood Federation.

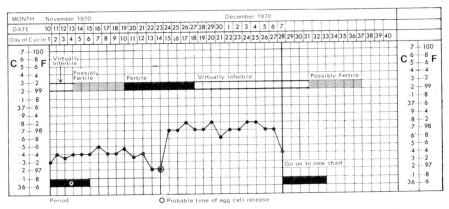

Fig. 14.3. A specimen temperature chart of a 28-day cycle.

PROGESTERONE PILL

The progesterone pill or mini pill does not suppress ovulation, it acts on cervical mucus making it thick and impenetrable to sperm. It also affects the uterine tubes and endometrium, making these areas unreceptive. It is a less effective contraceptive than combined oestrogen and progesterone but is recommended for women who cannot tolerate oestrogens. There are far less serious side effects with the progesterone only pill, but *breakthrough* bleeding or *spotting* makes the mini pill unacceptable to many women. The progesterone only pill must be taken diligently at the same time each day to be effective.

Prevention of ovulation

The combined pill of oestrogen and progesterone suppresses ovulation by mimicking the negative feedback mechanism to the pituitary gland and hypothalamus, inhibiting secretion of the gonadotrophic hormones. The ovarian cycle is largely suppressed so that ovarian follicles are not ripened, ovulation does not take place, and the endometrium is not prepared for implantation. A course of pills is taken for 21 days with a 7-day interval in between courses. Bleeding which occurs in the pill free interval is not true menstruation and usually only lasts for 2-3 days. There are many advantages and disadvantages (some serious) which must be considered with this method of contraception, bearing in mind that the pill is the most effective method of contraception.

ADVANTAGES

Many women have their psychological stability disrupted by the constant fear of becoming pregnant. The pill can remove this fear and is highly effective (99 %) if used in accordance with instructions. Menstrual irregularities such as prolonged and heavy bleeding are often improved by oral contraceptives. Endometriosis may become quiescent in women who regularly take the pill and relief from premenstrual tension may be obtained.

DISADVANTAGES

Many of the disadvantages or side effects of the combined pill can be minimized if factors such as age, cigarette smoking, obesity and oestrogen dosage are taken into account. Minor side effects which are not life-threatening may be very disturbing for women and include:
Breakthrough bleeding
Loss of libido
Weight gain
Cervical erosion (pill ectopy)
Nausea
Migraine

Chloasma
Altered tolerance to contact lenses
Major side effects which involve some serious diseases are:
Deep vein thrombosis
Pulmonary embolism
Cerebral thrombosis
Hypertension

Women who take oral contraceptives may suffer severe depression or mood changes, and may experience disorders of the gall bladder and the liver. Before the pill is prescribed a full medical history will be taken and a clinical examination performed. Many doctors advise discontinuation of the pill for 6 weeks prior to surgery because of the risk of postoperative thromboembolic disease. It is important to note that antibiotics render the pill ineffective, by causing gastrointestinal tract upsets and diarrhoea.

After a woman stops taking the pill ovulation may be delayed for months and in some cases years resulting in post-pill amenorrhoea.

Prevention of implantation

INTRAUTERINE CONTRACEPTIVE DEVICE (IUCD)

The term intrauterine device, abbreviated IUD may possibly be confusing and taken to mean intrauterine death. This misunderstanding is avoided by referring to it as an intrauterine contraceptive device and using the abbreviation IUCD.

The mode of action of intrauterine contraceptive devices is uncertain. It may be that peristalsis of the uterine tubes is increased causing the ova to be rushed along the tube too quickly. It is known that an inflammatory response is provoked in the endometrium which prevents implantation. This inflammatory response is similar to that provoked by a foreign body. Intrauterine contraceptive devices are made of plastic or a combination of plastic and copper. A sample of types available is shown in figure 14.4. Copper acts as an antifertility agent which is released slowly over a period of 2-3 years.

The Lippes loop and the Saf-T coil are the larger, plastic devices which can be left in the uterus for many years. Copper devices are smaller and cause less excessive bleeding but because the copper deteriorates they need more frequent replacement. The choice of device depends upon the stage of reproductive life reached.

Insertion

Uterine contraceptive devices are best inserted immediately following a menstrual period, this confirms that a pregnancy has not occurred already. A full medical social and gynaecological history will be taken before insertion.

The IUCD is loaded into a special introducer using full aseptic technique. This procedure which is usually done in an outpatient clinic requires the patient

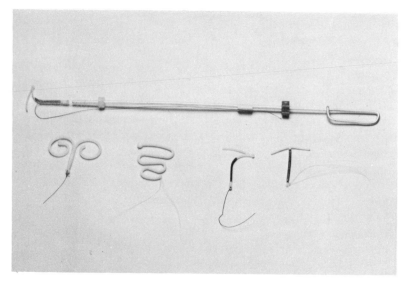

Fig. 14.4. Intrauterine contraceptive devices and applicator.

being placed in the lithotomy position. A general anaesthesia is seldom necessary.

The loaded introducer is inserted into the cervical canal and the plunger depressed so that the IUCD is delivered into the uterine cavity, leaving nylon threads visible through the cervix (Fig. 14.5). These threads are then trimmed with sterile scissors. The patient is returned to the dorsal position and allowed to rest for a short while. Before being sent home she is taught how to locate the threads in the vagina so that the presence of the device is confirmed. Preferably this should be done after each period. Followup is usually arranged 1 month after insertion.

Among the adverse effects of the IUCD are menorrhagia, dysmenorrhoea and intermenstrual bleeding. Perforation may occur at the time of insertion and expulsion of the IUCD can take place especially at the time of menstruation. Pelvic infection and pelvic inflammatory disease are more likely in women with an IUCD *in situ*.

The advantages are that it is an alternative method of contraception for women for whom the pill is contraindicated, or who find other methods unacceptable. The device has an effectiveness of approximately 98 %. Intrauterine contraceptive devices are easily removed by applying firm steady traction to the nylon threads. Occasionally the threads may not be visible as they may have retreated up into the uterus and have to be retrieved by using a fine plastic helix.

Other forms of contraception

Research at present is concentrating on other forms of contraception including the *morning-after* pill. This is a form of postcoital contraception which depends

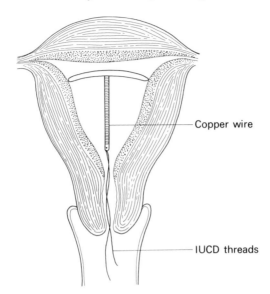

Copper wire

IUCD threads

Fig. 14.5. A copper 'T' IUCD *in situ*.

upon high dosages of oestrogen being taken within 24-72 hours of unprotected sexual intercourse. Work is being carried out on a male oral contraceptive which works by suppressing spermatogenesis. Recently trials have been carried out by some family planning authorities on a progesterone impregnated vaginal ring, which renders the cervical mucus hostile to sperm and the endometrium unreceptive. These methods have yet to be evaluated with regard to their safety and effectiveness.

Research into long-acting, slow-release hormone preparations continues and it may not be too long before a once a month or even once a year pill is marketed. Already in use is a preparation called medroxyprogesterone (Depo-Provera) given by a single intramuscular injection which is repeated at 3-monthly intervals. The main disadvantages of Depo-Provera are that it is not entirely reliable and may cause irregular bleeding at first but in time amenorrhoea.

STERILIZATION

After completing her family a woman may well have two decades or more of fertile life before the menopause. For this reason she may opt for a more permanent method of contraception, an elective sterilization. This is a surgical technique which may be done through a laparotomy incision or through a laparoscope or by the vaginal route.

Laparoscopic sterilization is becoming increasingly popular, it is a relatively simple surgical procedure with minimal side effects. Preoperative counselling is important, women must be assured that sexual activity will not be affected in any way and that the hormonal cycle will remain unaltered. Couples must look upon sterilization as permanent. In some cases reversal operations can be carried out but pregnancy cannot be guaranteed. Similarly an absolute guarantee that sterilization will be 100 % effective cannot be given. Written consent should be obtained from both husband and wife.

In the laparotomy method a piece of the middle part of each uterine tube is excised and the severed ends ligated. Some gynaecologists then bury the ligatured ends of each tube in the broad ligament.

Laparoscopic sterilization

The quick and simple operation of laparoscopic sterilization is becoming more popular. The peritoneal cavity is firstly inflated with CO_2 so that a pneumo-peritoneum is created. The laparoscope is then inserted through a small umbilical incision. Once pelvic structures are visualized through the laparoscope coagulation diathermy can be applied to both uterine tubes. Because diathermy can create burns and damage to nearby structures it is largely being replaced by the application of plastic rings or clips which occlude each uterine tube. This procedure creates minimal scarring and reduces the time spent in hospital to approximately 48 hours.

Male sterilization

A vasectomy can be performed under local anaesthetic as an outpatient pro-cedure. As with female sterilization preoperative counselling is important. The procedure involves small bilateral scrotal incisions through which the vas deferens is identified. Small segments are then removed from each vas deferens and the ends ligatured. The operation is not immediately effective as sperm remains in the semen for some time. Semen must be tested after intervals of 3 and 4 months to confirm that it is free of spermatazoa. The number of ejacu-lations is obviously a relevant factor.

15 Health Education and Screening

Gynaecology as with all branches of medicine is concerned with prevention and early detection of disease or abnormality. Screening procedures may be carried out at various stages of reproductive life, and during pregnancy. Many towns have developed the concept of preventative medicine and created *Well Women Clinics*. These clinics provide for women of all social classes but specifically cater for women in high risk social groups.

SCREENING IN PREGNANCY

A diagnosis can be made with greater accuracy with screening during pregnancy and allows counselling to take place when findings are known.

Radiological examination is done much less often these days as there is a small risk to the fetus. Ultrasound techniques, which are continually improving, are largely replacing X-ray examination.

Ultrasonography

Ultrasound is the production of a sound frequency which is too high to be heard by the human ear. Beams of ultrasound are directed from the equipment via a transducer towards an organ such as the uterus or other pelvic structure. Because of the density of solid tissue these beams are reflected back to the equipment where they visually depict on a screen the internal organs at which they had been aimed. The more dense or solid the structure the sharper the definition of the reflected beams become so that a clear picture (sonogram) emerges.

Real-time ultrasound scanning (ultrasonography) simply means that screen images are created of tissues as they exist at that point in time, i.e., an instantaneous image. Fetal viability, fetal death and missed abortion can all be detected by ultrasound scanning techniques. Ultrasound fetal heart detectors such as Sonicaid which make use of the Doppler effect produce an audio signal and are useful diagnostic aids if fetal death is suspected. Other uses of ultrasound scanning include the diagnosis of an ectopic pregnancy, a hydatidiform mole, a multiple pregnancy, the gestational age of the fetus, and neural tube defects. Diagnosis of ovarian and uterine tumours can be confirmed by ultrasound techniques.

PREPARATION OF THE PATIENT

Psychological preparation of the patient must take place as naturally her emotions will be mixed. She will be both hopeful and anxious, and the nurse must understand the reason why the scan is being performed and what the possible outcome might be. Before the procedure the bladder *must* be full. This brings the uterus into the abdominal cavity and displaces bowel structure, improving visualization.

On completion oil which will have been applied to the abdomen must be removed and the patient allowed to empty her bladder. As a general rule when the result is known the patient should be informed.

Amniocentesis

Amniocentesis may be performed by passing a needle into the amniotic cavity and withdrawing a small quantity of fluid for analysis. It is a diagnostic procedure which is usually performed between the fourteenth and eighteenth week of pregnancy. An ultrasound scan is performed as a preliminary to amniocentesis so that puncture of the fetus, placenta or cord is avoided. The risk of abortion after amniocentesis is estimated to be 1-2 %.

The amniotic fluid is examined for:
   Chromosomal abnormalities
   Alphafetoprotein
   Cell morphology
   Biochemical factors

Conditions such as Down's syndrome, neural tube defects, i.e., spina bifida, anencephaly, and other types of fetal deformity or disease may be detected by this examination. In neural tube defects the alphafetoprotein is increased in amount due to leakage from the fetus. When amniocentesis is performed in late pregnancy (32 weeks) antibodies may be discovered which indicate erythrocyte destruction (fetal haemolysis) is taking place. Exchange transfusion is necessary in this case.

TECHNIQUE

Amniocentesis is made comparatively safe by using an aseptic technique and performing an ultrasound scan prior to the procedure. The bladder must be emptied just before amniocentesis.

After the procedure rest should be allowed for approximately 1 hour and refreshment should be provided. Observations must be made for the onset of contractions and any leakage of liquor must be reported immediately. Since amniocentesis is often performed with the object of terminating an abnormal pregnancy, it is essential that psychological care is given throughout.

The nurse must be aware that the patient may display shock and even anger and that these are important emotional responses. The delay in awaiting results in each screening method may intensify stress and anxiety, this is particularly so in amniocentesis as a lengthy technical process is needed before the results are known. The nurse should be able to tell the patient the approximate lengths of time she will have to wait for results, i.e., some biochemical results may be available in 3 days, chromosomal studies in 3 weeks.

Fetoscopy

Not all fetal deformities are discovered by ultrasound scan or amniocentesis. The fetus may not be leaking alphafetoprotein. Direct visualization of the fetus through a fibreoptic endoscope (fetoscopy) may reveal deformities not easily detected by other prenatal screening methods. Fetal blood can also be obtained by this method and tested for genetic abnormalities which may not be revealed by amniocentesis. Fetoscopy however is a very specialized technique which requires a high degree of skill. The risk of miscarriage following fetoscopy is at present estimated at 5-10 %.

Genetic counselling

Prenatal diagnosis is advancing rapidly. Ultrasonic scanning, fetoscopy and fetal blood and tissue sampling are techniques which are likely to be refined in the near future. When genetic disorders are discovered they are rarely curable, therefore provision has to be made for a genetic counselling service. These departments are now being established in many hospitals.

The diagnosis of a particular disorder will allow the geneticist to predict inheritance patterns and risks to future pregnancies. Families have to be advised with tact, sympathy and understanding yet ultimately when all the relevant predictions have been made, make their own decisions. A large part of a genetic counsellor's work is concerned with helping couples and families to come to terms with and adjust to abnormality.

WELL WOMEN CLINICS

In the early 1980s several health authorities established clinics which they hoped would meet the specific needs of women with regard to health problems. Community health councils in many areas were initially responsible for submitting proposals and formulating the aims and objectives for Well Women Clinics. These broadly are:

To meet specific health needs of women.

To provide a greater awareness of the health of the individual and the agencies available which provide health care.

To provide an alternative to general practitioner consultation.

Well Women Clinics hope to attract groups of women who traditionally have avoided visiting their doctors or were unaware of services available and have therefore become high risk groups. The overall aim of these clinics is the prevention and early diagnosis of disease.

Staff who work in these clinics are able to spend much more time with patients than the general practitioner can usually afford. In this way intimate problems may be discussed at length and advice given. It may emerge from discussion that marriage guidance might be helpful or that psychosexual counselling is needed. If simple screening tests reveal any abnormality the woman will be referred to her general practitioner. Particular attention is paid to conditions related to premenstrual tension, the menopause, health in relationship to diet, and urogenital problems.

Several clinics ask women to complete an optional confidential questionnaire which includes a wide range of questions on physical and psychosocial matters. What women seen to value most of all is the time made available for discussion. They also appreciate the fact that most of the staff are women who can fully appreciate female difficulties and problems. These newly established clinics are in the process of being evaluated as to their effectiveness in meeting the needs of attenders and whether they are achieving their aim of attracting women in previously identified high risk groups.

BREAST SCREENING

Breast self-examination, mammography and thermography are methods of breast screening.

Breast self-examination

Breast examination is an integral part of the gynaecological examination process. Family Planning and Well Women Clinics take the opportunity to teach the women who attend how to examine their own breast through breast self-examination (BSE). It is an easy technique which can be performed during bathing or at some other suitable time. The woman is taught to examine her breasts regularly preferably just after menstruation each month.

Using the flat of one hand she is taught how to palpate the upper, lower and central aspects of each breast. She is taught to examine the axillae in the same way. Visual examination is also advised; the woman stands in front of a mirror with both arms by her side and looks carefully for any changes in the contour of her breasts: any swellings, dimpling or retraction of the nipple should be noted. The exercise is repeated, this time standing with her arms above her head. The limitations of BSE must be appreciated.

It is unlikely that any tumour less than 1 cm in diameter will be discovered by this method. Any lesion greater than 1 cm presents a poor prognosis. However a tumour discovered by this method is at least treated when it is small.

Mammography

A technique which uses soft tissue radiography (mammography) can distinguish between tumours and inflammatory changes. It is particularly useful for patients in high risk groups or in whom breast examination is difficult. Mammography is a diagnostic tool which could be available for mass screening programmes, however the cost effectiveness of such a community project must be considered. In a recent feasibility study it emerged that of 3,000 women screened 70 lesions were found and of these 9 malignant tumours diagnosed. With economic recession many countries cannot launch a national screening programme though intensive public education projects can be mounted at far less cost.

Thermography

With thermography tumours are detected by measuring infra-red heat emission from the breast. Abnormal tissue emits more heat, so that tumours can be detected which were not palpable.

CERVICAL CYTOLOGY

The method of obtaining a cervical smear has been outlined in chapter 2. A brief review, however, of cervical cytology as a screening procedure is needed as in recent years there has been an increase in the number of deaths from carcinoma of the cervix in young women.

Cervical cytology has not resulted in the elimination of cervical cancer because mass screening has not reached the 'at risk' groups. This means cases have not been diagnosed early enough. This may be due to the fact that too few women attend for cervical smears and that once again the high risk groups (social classes 4-5) do not attend and are overlooked.

An intensive programme of cervical cytology has to be undertaken if cervical cancer is to be irradicated. There is existing evidence to show that in parts of the world where intensive screening is done the incidence of cervical cancer has markedly declined. Health education councils can play a vital part in promoting cervical cytology and establishing a pattern of early and regular cytology. Wide publication is essential and rather than relying upon an individual's initiative to attend clinic perhaps a system could be devised in which invitations were sent out to encourage attendance.

TOXIC SHOCK SYNDROME

Toxic shock syndrome (TSS) is a newly recognized disease which was first described in 1978 in the United States. It is an uncommon disease the pathogenesis of which is uncertain. It affects apparently healthy women and is associated with the use of tampons, in fact in 90 % of the reported cases of TSS tampons had been used.

Vaginal and cervical cultures usually reveal the presence of *Staphylococcus aureus* which evidently produces a toxin. The onset of the disease is sudden and almost always during or just after menses. Symptoms include vomiting, diarrhoea, headache, abdominal pain, sore throat, hypotension and oliguria. There is typically a pyrexia of more than 38°C. Other systems may be affected or vague symptoms may also be present. There may be a erythematous rash.

Some cases of toxic shock syndrome are relatively mild and may be self-limiting, others may result in the woman being shocked with a lowered central venous pressure and oliguria. In this profound version admission to an intensive care unit is advisable. Priorities of treatment are as follows:

Removal of tampon

Intravenous fluid replacement

Commencement of antibiotic therapy

Monitoring of renal function

The nursing care of the patient must be equally intensive.

It is impractical to expect women to stop using tampons but they must be urged to change them frequently and alternate with other methods of protection. Hygiene must be scrupulous during the menstrual period. Some packets of tampons carry a warning about TSS and suggest a few precautions which tampon users must bear in mind.

Health education councils can play a vital part in making the public aware of this new hazard and schools should make sure that menstruating adolescents appreciate the situation regarding the use of tampons.

16 Gynaecological Theatre

The preparation of a gynaecological theatre is essentially the same as for general surgery. The essentials of preoperative and postoperative care have already been outlined at the beginning of this book. In this chapter a brief description of some of the instruments and equipment used is intended plus a brief summary of the common gynaecological operations.

PREPARATION OF THE PATIENT

Any nurse escorting a patient to the operating theatre must be aware of the anxiety and psychological stress which her patient may be under. All patients experience stress prior to operative procedures, gynaecological patients go to the operating theatre sometimes in the knowledge that their reproductive function will be affected and with the feeling that their femininity may be altered.

It is a mistake to force a woman to listen to information she has no wish to hear and there is a danger in gynaecology of regarding natural emotional responses as grave psychological problems. Sometimes patients simply need time and understanding before they adjust. The skilled nurse will soon recognize those patients who require additional help.

It is part of nursing responsibility to make sure that the patient understands the nature of the proposed surgery, and what she might expect to find in the way of drainage tubes, intravenous lines, vaginal pack etc. when she recovers from anaesthesia. Checking that written consent has been obtained is particularly important in gynaecological surgery.

CONDITIONS OF CONSENT

Operations which affect fertility generally require the signature of husband and wife on the consent form. The husband's consent is not *legally* necessary but the law is unclear on the position if sterilization is carried out for a *non-medical reason*. It appears that there could be grounds for legal action in this case if the husband has not been consulted previously.

For termination of pregnancy the woman's consent only is needed but if circumstances permit the husband will be consulted. The legal age of consent in Great Britain is 16 years and over, parental consent is therefore unnecessary.

TYPES OF INSTRUMENT

Instruments used in gynaecological surgery include an abdominal set, a dilatation and curettage set, and a laparoscope.

Abdominal set

A typical abdominal set (Fig. 16.1) will be prepared with:

    4 Rampley's sponge-holding forceps
    3 Toothed forceps—Waugh's, Bonney's and plain
    10 Cairns' curved artery forceps
    10 Spencer Wells straight artery forceps
    2 Spencer Wells artery forceps—25 cm
    5 Curved Spencer Wells artery forceps
    2 Vulsellum forceps
    5 Heaney's artery forceps
    3 Mayo-Hegar needle holders
    5 Littlewood's tissue forceps
    1 Morris box retractor
    1 Doyen's pelvic retractor with chain (weight not shown)
    2 Bard-Parker handles (Number 4)
    1 Mayo curved scissors
    1 blunt-ended scissors
    1 Ferguson's scissors
    5 Cross action towel clips

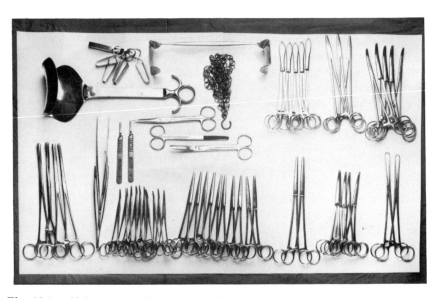

Fig. 16.1.   Abdominal set of gynaecological instruments.

Dilatation and curettage set

A typical dilatation and curettage (D & C) set (Fig. 16.2) will include:

    7 Graduated Hegar's dilators
    2 Vulsellum forceps

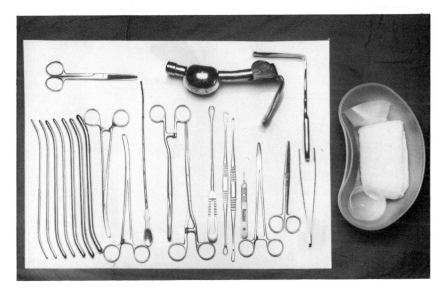

Fig. 16.2. A dilatation and curettage set of instruments.

1 Uterine sound
1 Rampley's sponge-holding forceps
1 Ovum forceps
1 Blunt curette
1 Sharp curette
1 Double-ended curette
1 Bard-Parker handle (Number 3)
1 Mayo-Hegar needle holder
1 Mayo straight blunt scissors
1 Bonney's toothed forceps
1 Angled vaginal retractor
1 Auvard speculum
1 Blunt scissors

Laparoscope

The fibreoptic instrument through which the pelvic contents and other abdominal organs can be directly visualized is known as a laparoscope (Fig. 16.3a). Surgical procedures such as sterilization and ovarian biopsy may be carried out through the operating laparoscope. A photolaparoscope enables photographs of pelvic organs to be taken. With the anaesthetized patient in the lithotomy position the bladder is catheterized. Then the cervix is grasped with a Vulsellum forceps so that the uterus can be manipulated during the procedure. Next a pneumoperitoneum is created by distending the abdomen, with approximately 3-4 litres of carbon dioxide via a Verres needle. Through a small incision a large

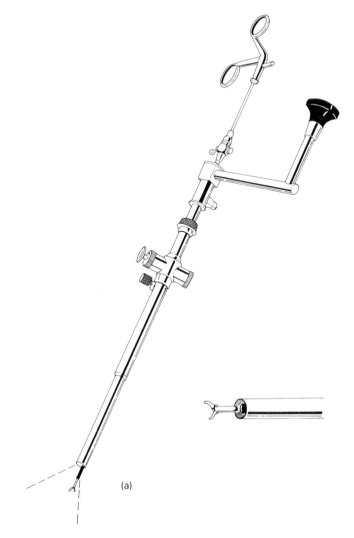

Fig. 16.3. (a) A laparoscope.

trocar and cannula is inserted just below the umbilicus, the trocar is replaced by the laparoscope. Once in position the laparoscope can be manipulated to obtain a view of all the pelvic organs. Surgical procedures may be performed through another cannula (Fig. 16.3b).

POSITIONS

In the theatre, the patient may be placed in a modified Trendelenburg or in the lithotomy position.

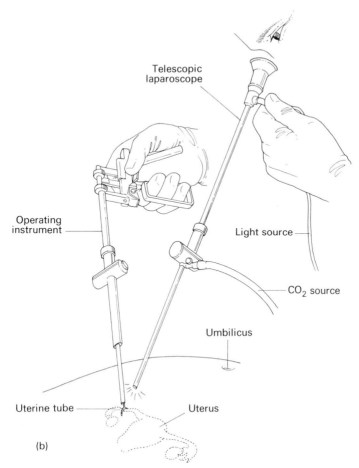

Telescopic laparoscope

Operating instrument

Light source

CO_2 source

Umbilicus

Uterine tube

Uterus

(b)

Fig. 16.3. (b) An operating instrument coupled with laparoscope enables tubal surgery to be performed.

Modified Trendelenburg

For operations on the pelvic cavity the modified Trendelenburg position is usually used. The operating table is tilted so that the patient's head is several degrees lower than her feet (Fig. 16.4). The patient is safely retained in position by a corrugated ribbed (non-slip) mattress. Gravity displaces the intestines towards the upper abdomen allowing easier access to the pelvic organs.

Lithotomy

The position used in gynaecological surgery for vulval, vaginal and perineal operations is the lithotomy position (see Fig. 2.2d). Both stirrup poles at the end of the operating table must be carefully adjusted to the same height and should be padded for protection. Two nurses must lift the patient's legs *simultaneously*,

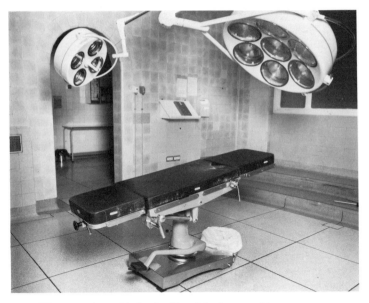

Fig. 16.4. The operating table in the Trendelenberg position.

flexing them then abducting them and securing them in the foot stirrups on the *outside* of each pole. The patient's legs must be lifted simultaneously so that sacroiliac strain is avoided. Abduction of the legs ensures that venous return of blood is maintained.

With both positions care must be taken of the patient's arms. The nurse must position and secure both arms across the chest or on armboards. Alternatively arm retainers may be used.

OPERATIONS AND PROCEDURES

Various operations and procedures are carried out in the gynaecological theatre; those usually referred to as 'minor' commonly include dilatation and curettage, cautery of the cervix, evacuation of the uterus and biopsy of the cervix. Common 'major' operations include hysterectomy and colporrhaphy.

Operations and procedures are performed through one of the following routes: vaginal, vulval or abdominal. Surgery performed via the abdomen may involve one of the following incisions, midline, paramedian or Pfannenstiel. The Pfannenstiel is a transverse lower abdominal incision which follows the suprapubic crease.

Examination under anaesthesia

Pelvic examination under general anaesthesia (EUA) becomes necessary for patients in the following circumstances: The patient with an *intact hymen* who would find vaginal examination intolerable. The patient who finds it physically *impossible to relax* her pelvic and abdominal muscles and the patient who has an excessive amount of *abdominal fat* thus making bimanual examination unsatisfactory. It is also necessary for patients in whom examination without anaesthesia has proved *inconclusive.*

Dilatation and curettage

The cervix is dilated with graduated cervical dilators (see Fig. 16.2) and then endometrial tissue obtained by curette. This procedure may be *diagnostic,* to confirm malignant disease or other endometrial pathology or it may be *therapeutic* in conditions such as menorrhagia or dysmenorrhoea.

Cautery of the cervix

Cauterization is performed for erosions of the cervix. Cautery and diathermy both destroy tissue lesions by the application of intense heat. More extensive lesions are treated by these methods. Milder lesions may be treated by cryosurgery which is the application of intense cold. A cryoprobe is used to freeze cervical lesions, it is a procedure which may be carried out in an outpatient department.

Evacuation of the uterus

With the anaesthetized patient in the lithotomy position evacuation of the uterus is performed when the products of conception are retained in the uterus following abortion. Cervical dilatation may not be necessary and the uterus is emptied by sponge-holding forceps or a sharp curette. The doctor will then insert a gloved finger into the uterus to confirm that the uterine cavity is completely empty. Evacuation of the uterus may be carried out for missed abortion. *Note* some gynaecologists consider it safer to use a blunt curette.

Biopsy of the cervix

Once a surface lesion has been identified small biopsies of cervical tissue can be obtained by *punch biopsy* forceps. A much more extensive biopsy is the *cone biopsy.* This consists of the removal of a cone-shaped piece of tissue from around the cervical canal (see chap. 8). Histological examination will reveal whether or not the whole of the abnormal tissue has been removed. Remember that haemorrhage can be severe following a cone biopsy.

The uterus

Uterine operations may involve removing the uterus, and to varying degrees the surrounding tissue, or may involve correcting the position of the uterus.

ABDOMINAL HYSTERECTOMY

In abdominal hysterectomy the uterine vessels are divided after curved Kocher's forceps have been placed across the base of the broad ligament. The vagina is opened with a scalpel anteriorly (Fig. 16.5a). The uterosacral ligaments are divided after securing them with Moynihan forceps, with one blade inserted intravaginally below the attachment of the cervix (Fig. 16.5b). The uterus is then removed (Fig. 16.5c) with the help of vulsellum forceps.

Total hysterectomy

A total hysterectomy consists of the removal of the body and the cervix of the uterus (Fig. 16.6a). This is often carried out for benign diseases of the uterus, e.g., menorrhagia, uterine myomata (fibroids). A vaginal hysterectomy is discussed under the section on vaginal operations.

Subtotal hysterectomy

The body of the uterus is removed but the cervix is not when a subtotal hysterectomy is performed (Fig. 16.6b). This may be because of technical difficulties, e.g., extensive fibrous tissue making surgical dissection difficult.

Extended hysterectomy

A total hysterectomy with bilateral salpingo-öophorectomy and removal of the cuff of the vagina is known as an extended hysterectomy (Fig. 16.6c). This operative procedure is undertaken for patients with a malignant condition. The cuff of the vagina is removed because the vault is a common site of recurrence.

Wertheim's hysterectomy

A Wertheim's hysterectomy is an extended hysterectomy with the additional removal of the pelvic connective tissue, lymph nodes and the upper one third of the vagina. (The ovaries *may* be conserved in some younger women.)

Pelvic exenteration (*total*)

In younger women with advanced carcinoma of the cervix who are fit to withstand extensive surgery, pelvic exenteration is sometimes undertaken. All of the pelvic organs are removed. This includes Wertheim's hysterectomy with total cystectomy and transplantation of the ureters into an ileal loop, excision of the rectum and formation of a colostomy. Some authorities are of the opinion that such extensive surgery is hard to justify.

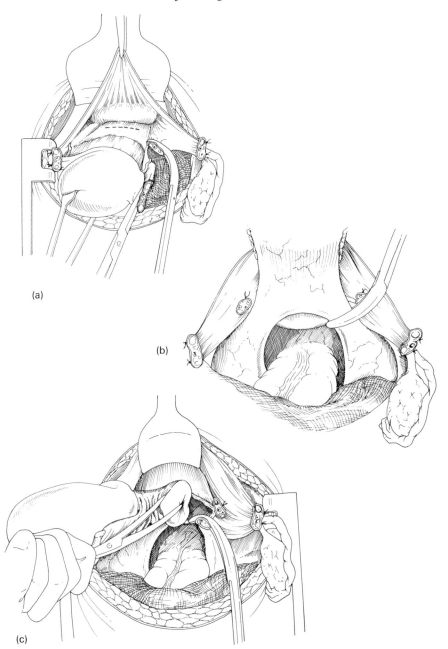

(a)

(b)

(c)

Fig. 16.5. An abdominal hysterectomy: the vagina is opened with a scalpel (a), the uterosacral ligaments are divided (b), the uterus is removed (c). (Produced by permission of Ethicon Ltd *Trademark © Ethicon Ltd 1982.)

Gilliam's ventrosuspension operation consists of drawing a loop of the round ligament from each side of the uterus and suturing both loops together on the anterior rectus sheath. Alternatively the round ligaments may be plicated (pleated) with a suture. This operation is carried out to correct the position of the uterus.

The uterine tubes

Uterine tube operations are aimed at restoring tubal patency. In *salpingostomy* the uterine tube is opened at the fimbrial end. A cuff may be turned back and sutured. Patency following this procedure is maintained by a polythene *splint*

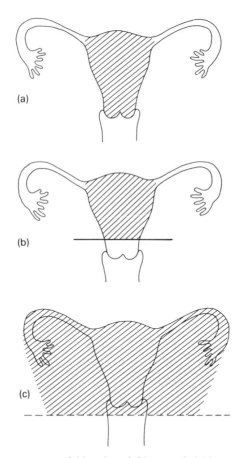

Fig. 16.6. Hysterectomy: total (a), subtotal (b), extended (c).

which is passed through the tube, into the uterine cavity and out through the cervix. This splint remains in position for several weeks. *Salpingoloysis* consists of freeing the tube by dividing peritubal adhesions. *Salpingectomy*, removal of a tube (Fig. 16.7), is performed for conditions such as ectopic pregnancy, chronic salpinitis or malignant disease.

The ovaries

In *oöphorectomy* the whole of the ovary is removed usually for conditions such as malignant tumours, cysts which are too large to excise and chronic infections. *Ovarian cystectomy* is the removal of the cyst alone. Wedge *resection* of the ovary is occasionally carried out to treat polycystic ovary disease, but modern drug therapy is more often used to correct the endocrine imbalance these days.

The vulva

Vulval operations include a simple vulvectomy and a radical vulvectomy, and the excision, drainage or marsupialization of the Bartholin's gland (see chap. 6).

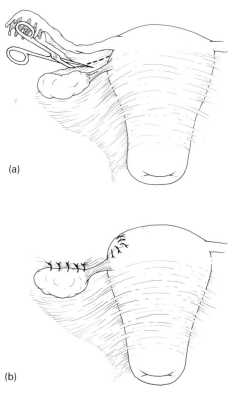

(a)

(b)

Fig. 16.7. Salpingectomy: the broad ligaments are divided (a), the uterine tube is removed and the ovary is left intact (b).

The vagina

Vaginal operations include anterior and posterior colporrhaphy (see section on Prolapse, chap. 8) and the repair of fistulae (see chap. 6). Vaginal reconstruction may be undertaken for congenital abnormality and vaginectomy carried out in malignant disease.

Manchester repair

In Manchester repair the anterior and posterior vaginal walls are excised. The operation is performed with the patient in the lithotomy position. After cleaning and draping the vulval area, the bladder may be catheterized. (Some surgeons prefer to leave the bladder full which makes separation from the vaginal skin easier.) For anterior repair, the incision is in the anterior vaginal wall, encircling the cervix posteriorly (Fig. 16.8a). The vaginal skin is peeled back and the bladder pushed anteriorly (Fig. 16.8b). The uterosacral ligaments are transfixed and following their bilateral division, the cervix is amputated (Fig. 16.8c). When the cervix has been amputated, the stump is covered by peritoneum using the Sturmdorf suture technique (Fig. 16.8d). The perineal body muscles are sutured using deep interrupted stitches (Fig. 16.8e) and the perineal skin in closed with interrupted or subcuticular stitches (Fig. 16.8f).

VAGINAL HYSTERECTOMY

One advantage of removing the uterus via a vaginal route is that abdominal scarring is avoided. The uterus is removed after the broad, round and ovarian ligaments are clamped and divided (see fig. 16.9). The tubes and ovaries may or may not require removal. The pedicles of the ligaments are sutured together so as to afford support and a repair operation is usually combined with this procedure.

DRUGS IN GYNAECOLOGICAL THEATRE

Apart from the usual drugs used to induce anaesthesia and those used to combat shock or relieve pain, it is essential to ensure adequate supplies of oxytocin or ergometrine or both. These drugs act directly on the uterus controlling haemorrhage, e.g., following incomplete abortion. Syntometrine, a combination of ergometrine maleate 500 μg and oxytocin 5 units, may be given intramuscularly. Intravenous synthetic oxytocin (Syntocinon) may also be effective in controlling uterine haemorrhage.

When the patient has fully recovered from the effects of anaesthesia a full explanation should be given of the operation performed, which structures have been removed and which structures remain behind. It is important that the patient fully understands the physiological effects of surgery and knows what to expect when she goes home.

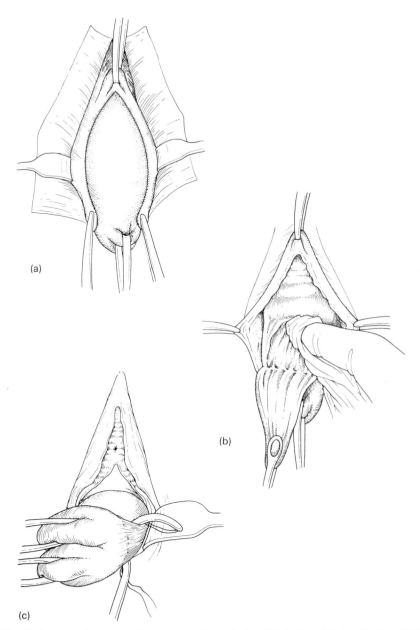

(a)

(b)

(c)

Fig. 16.8. Manchester repair operation: the vaginal wall is incised (a), the skin is pulled back (b), the cervix is amputated (c).

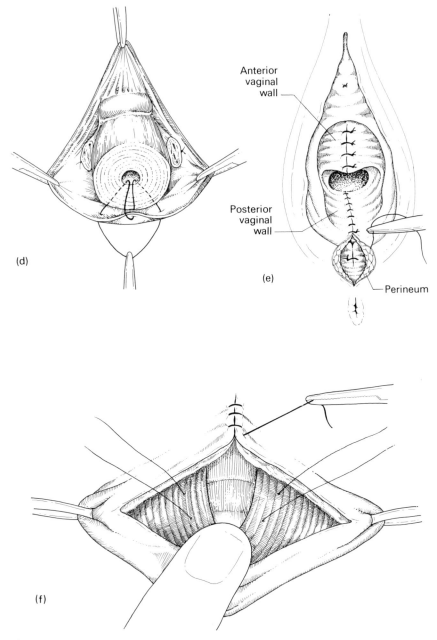

Fig. 16.8. (*cont*).   The cervix is covered with vaginal skin (d), the perineal muscles are sutured (e), the perineal skin is closed (f). (Produced by permission of Ethicon Ltd *Trademark © Ethicon Ltd 1982.)

Some surgeons believe that the patient is more reassured if she is allowed to see histological reports which confirm normality before she is discharged from hospital.

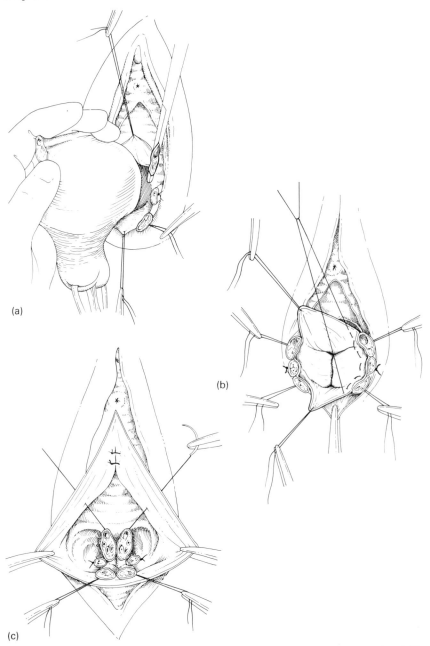

Fig. 16.9. Vaginal hysterectomy: the uterus is removed (a), the peritoneum is closed (b), the round ligaments are sutured for support (c). (Produced by permission of Ethicon Ltd *Trademark © Ethicon Ltd 1982.)

Glossary

The language of gynaecology seems at first to be both strange and difficult. The prefix to many words is Latin or Greek. The following glossary contains most of the common terms used in gynaecology and should be useful for quick reference.

Abortion Cessation of pregnancy before the twenty-eighth week when the fetus is said to be viable, i.e., capable of an independent existence. In other parts of the world this is 20 weeks but in the UK this is 28 weeks.

Adenomyosis Endometrial tissue found in the uterine muscle as well as in its usual location in the uterine cavity.

Adnexae Tissue either side of the uterus, i.e., uterine tubes and ovaries.

Amenorrhoea Absence of menstruation.

Androgen Masculizing hormone.

Appendages See *adnexae*.

Atrophy Decrease in the size of normally developed tissues or organs.

Ayre's smear Cytological test for diagnosing an abnormality of the cervix, e.g., pre-invasive carcinoma.

Barr bodies In genetic females, a small mass of chromatin found on the nuclear membrane.

Bicornuate Uterus with two horns.

Buttressing Strengthening of tissues and structures. In gynaecology it is the urethra which requires a buttress operation.

Carneous mole Fleshy mole containing old, firm bloodclot, usually the outcome of a missed abortion.

Caruncle Small red fleshy nodule which is usually extremely tender.

Chancre Lesion resembling an ulcer associated with syphilis.

CIN Initials meaning cervical intraepithelial neoplasia. Now largely used instead of carcinoma *in situ*.

Climacteric Cessation of ovarian function with general regression of all genital organs. Usually incorrectly called the menopause which is only one feature of the climacteric.

Coitus Act of sexual intercourse; copulation.

Colpo Prefix denoting vagina.

Colporrhaphy Vaginal repair in which sutures are used.

Colpotomy Incision of the vaginal wall, usually the posterior vaginal vault.

Cone biopsy Wedge-shaped piece of tissue which is taken from the cervix. It is diagnostic in carcinoma of the cervix.

Conception Fertilization of the ovum by the spermatazoon; to become pregnant.

Corpus luteum Latin derivation; corpus meaning body, luteum meaning yellow. It is formed in the ovary after rupture of the Graafian follicle.

Cryptomenorrhoea Condition in which although there is menstruation the escape is prevented by an obstruction.

Culdoscopy Visualization of the contents of the pelvis through an incision in the vaginal wall into the pouch of Douglas.

Curettage Scraping of a cavity with a curette.

Cyesis Pregnancy.

Cystocele Prolapse and herniation of the urinary bladder caused by weakness of the anterior vaginal wall.

Cytology Study of cells especially for the detection of malignant cells.

Decidua Thickened lining of the uterus after fertilization has taken place. It may be shed after a miscarriage or an ectopic pregnancy.

Dermoid Made up of many different types of tissue, i.e., the dermoid cyst of the ovary which may contain bone, hair, etc.

Dyskaryosis Abnormality of the nuclei of cells.

Dysmenorrhoea Painful menstruation.

Dyspareunia Painful coitus.

Dysplasia Abnormal development or growth of cells.

Ectopic pregnancy Implantation of the fertilized ovum in any site other than the uterine cavity.

Embryo Early conceptus up until the eighth week following fertility.

Endocervix Mucous membrane lining of the cervical canal.

Endometriosis Ectopic endometrium which is found outside the uterine cavity.

Enterocele Usually a vaginal vault prolapse which contains intestines.

Episiotomy Incision of the perineum made during childbirth to avoid undue laceration.

Erosion Overgrowth of columnar epithelium around the external os.

Fetus The developing pregnancy from the ninth week of pregnancy to delivery.

Fertilization Fusion of the ovum and the spermatozoon.

Fibroid Benign tumour of the uterine muscle which contains fibrous tissue.

Fibromyomata See *fibroid*.

Fimbriae Finger-like projections of the distal end of the uterine tubes.

Fornix Recesses at the end of the vagina created by the downward projection of the cervix.

Fourchette Area of skin where the labia minora unite posteriorly.

Fundus Part of the uterus which lies above the insertion of the uterine tubes.

Genitalia Organs of reproduction.

Gestation Development of a pregnancy from conception to birth.

Gilliam's operation Specific operation which corrects retroversion by ventrosuspension.

Gonadatrophin Hormone which stimulates the gonads, i.e., ovaries and testes.

Graafian follicle Developed primary follicle which contains the ovum.

Gravida A pregnant woman.

Gravid Pregnant.

Haematocolpos Menstrual blood which collects in the vagina.

Hydatidiform mole Appearance of multiple small grape-like vessicles in the uterus.

Hydrosalpinx Uterine tube which is swollen with clear watery fluid in response to mild infection.

Hymen   Membrane guarding the entrance to the vagina.

Hyperemesis (gravidarum)   Excessive vomiting in pregnancy.

Hyperplasia   Increase in the size of organs or tissues.

Hysterectomy   Surgical removal of the uterus.

Hystero   Prefix pertaining to the uterus.

Hysteroscopy   Visualization of the uterine cavity.

Hysterotomy   Incision into the uterus; a method of termination of pregnancy.

Hysterosalpingography (HSG)   Radiography of the uterine cavity and uterine tubes. Diagnostic in tubal blockage.

Infertility   Inability to conceive.

Introitus   Entrance into the vagina.

Insemination   Introduction of male sperm into the female genital tract.

Insufflation   To blow air or gas into a cavity, usually the uterine tubes.

Kraurosis   Progressive atrophy of the vulva.

Lactation   Secretion of milk.

Laparoscopy   Visualization of the pelvic viscera and tissue through a laparoscope.

Leiomyomata   Benign muscular tumour, e.g., a fibroid.

Leucorrhoea   White vaginal discharge.

Leucoplakia   Thickened white patches on the vulva due to chronic inflammation and which may be premalignant.

Marsupialization   Drainage of a cyst, such as Bartholin's cyst, and suturing of the edges of the skin to the edges of the opened cavity.

Manchester operation (repair)   Repair of anterior and posterior vaginal walls with amputation of the cervix. The perineal muscle is also repaired.

Menarche   Establishment of menstrual periods usually at puberty.

Menopause   Cessation of menstrual periods usually at 45-50 years.

Menorrhagia   Excessive or prolonged bleeding at menstruation.

Menstruation Periodic shedding of blood, mucus and endometrial debris from the uterus usually at regular monthly intervals.

Mesovarium A fold of peritoneum connecting the broad ligament and the ovary.

Metaplasia Normal transformation of cellular tissue.

Metrorrhagia Irregular uterine bleeding not related to the normal menstrual cycle.

Multipara A woman who has had two or more children.

Myomectomy Surgical removal of fibroids.

Nullipara A woman who has never given birth to a child.

Oestrogen A hormone secreted by the Graafian follicle of the ovary.

Oöph Prefix pertaining to the ovary.

Oöphorectomy Removal of an ovary.

Os A mouth—the external and internal openings in the cervix.

Ovulation Production and release of an ova by the ovary.

Ovum Female egg cell.

Oxytocic An agent which contracts uterine muscle.

Papanicolaou Method of staining smears to detect malignant cells.

Parametrium Tissue lying to either side of and surrounding the uterus.

Parity Number of children a woman has borne.

Parturition Process of child birth.

Perineorrhophy Surgical repair of the perineum.

Placenta Afterbirth; a complex structure which provides nourishment for the developing fetus.

Pregnosticon Diagnostic test performed on urine to determine a pregnancy.

Procidentia Downward displacement especially of the uterus, when the neck of the uterus lies outside the vagina.

Products of conception All the elements of pregnancy, i.e., the embryo, membranes and placenta.

Prolapse Downward displacement of tissues or organs.

Pruritus Intense itching.

Pseudocyesis Phantom pregnancy.

Rectocele Prolapse and herniation of the rectum against a weakened vaginal wall.

Retroversion Backward displacement of the uterus.

Salpingectomy Removal of a uterine tube.

Salpingitis Inflammation of the uterine tubes.

Salpingolysis The breakdown of adhesions within and surrounding the uterine tube.

Salpingo-oöphorectomy Surgical removal of the uterine tube and an ovary.

Salpingostomy Surgical creation of an opening into the uterine tube.

Semen Fluid discharged from the penis (after being produced in the male reproductive organs).

Septate uterus Septum projecting downwards in the uterine cavity with the division of the uterus, cervix and vagina.

Shirodkar suture Suture which encircles the cervix and closes the cervical os.

Subseptate uterus Septum projecting downwards in the upper part of the uterus.

Trachelorrhaphy Repair of a lacerated cervix.

Trichomonas vaginalis Protozoal organism which infects the vagina.

Tubo-ovarian Denoting the uterine tube and ovary.

Unicornuate uterus Asymmetrical horn on one side of the uterus.

Urethrocele Prolapse of the urethra, against the anterior vaginal wall.

Urethroplasty Repair by plastic surgery of the urethra.

Urodynamic Movement of urine through the urinary tract.

Uterine didelphys Double uterus.

Vaginismus Strong, painful contractions of the muscles surrounding the vagina at intercourse.

Venereal   Transmitted by sexual intercourse.

Ventrosuspension   Shortening of the round ligaments in order to correct retroversion of the uterus.

Viability   Capable of a separate existence, i.e., of surviving independently.

Vulvectomy   Removal of the vulva.

References and Further Reading

Anderson M. (1983) *The Menopause*. London, Faber & Faber.

Barnes J. (1983) *Lecture Notes on Gynaecology*. 5th ed. Oxford, Blackwell Scientific Publications.

Bloom M. & Dongen L.V. (1972) *Clinical Gynaecology (Integration of Structure and Function)*. London, Heinemann.

British Society for Clinical Cytology (1981) *Taking Uterine Cervical Smears*. Aberdeen, University of Aberdeen Press.

Butterworths Medical Dictionary (1978) 2nd ed. Editor in Chief Macdonald Critchley. London, Butterworth. Excerpt reprinted by kind permission of Butterworths.

Catterall R.D. (1974) *A Short Textbook of Venerology*. London, The English Universities Press.

Catterall R.D. (1979) *Venereology and Genito-Urinary Medicine*. Sevenoaks, Kent, Hodder & Stoughton.

Cheetham J. (1977) *Unwanted Pregnancy and Counselling*. London, Routledge & Kegan Paul.

Clayton S.G. (1979) *A Pocket Gynaecology*. Edinburgh, Churchill Livingstone.

Cook R.J. & Senanayke P. (1978) *The Human Problem of Abortion (Medical and Legal Dimensions)*. London, IPPF.

The Concise Oxford Dictionary (1982) 7th ed. Edited by J.B. Sykes. Oxford, Oxford University Press. Excerpt reprinted by kind permission of Oxford University Press.

Cowper A. & Young S. (1981) *Fundamentals of Family Planning for Health Professionals*. London, Croom Helm.

Fraser H. (1979) *Gynaecological Care*, 1st ed. Tunbridge Wells, Kent, Pitman Medical.

Fream W.C. (1979) *Notes on Gynaecological Nursing*. Edinburgh, Churchill Livingstone.

Gardner R.S.G. (1975) *Abortion—The Personal Dilemma*. Exeter, The Paternoster Press.

Garrey M.W. *et al.* (1978) *Gynaecology Illustrated*, 2nd ed. Edinburgh, Churchill Livingstone.

Hawkins H.O.W. & Bourne G. (1971) *Shaw's Textbook of Gynaecology*, 9th ed. Edinburgh, Churchill Livingstone.

Hector W. (1980) *Modern Gynaecology with Obstetrics for Nurses*. London, Heinemann.

Hudson C.N. (1978) *The Female Reproductive System*. Edinburgh, Churchill Livingstone.

International Planned Parenthood Federation (1979) *Handbook of Infertility*. London, IPPF.

Johnson M.H. & Everitt B.J. (1980) *Essential Reproduction*. Oxford, Blackwell Scientific Publications.

Kolodny R.C. *et al.* (1979) *Textbook of Human Sexuality for Nurses*. Boston, Little Brown & Co.

Lees H. & Singer A. (1979) Operations for Malignant Disease, Vol. 3. London, Wolfe Medical.

Llewellyn-Jones D. (1978) *Everywoman: Gynaecological Guide for Life*, 2nd ed. London, Faber & Faber.

Llewellyn-Jones D. (1978) *Fundamentals of Gynaecology*, Vol. 2. London, Faber & Faber.

Manning M. (1982) Test-tube babies. A brave new world we could do without. *World Medicine*, Feb. p. 39.

Pinker G.D. & Roberts D.W.T. (1980) *Gynaecology and Obstetrics*. Sevenoaks, Kent, Hodder & Stoughton.

Reitz R. (1979) *The Menopause, A Positive Attitude*. Harmondsworth, Penguin Books.

Speck P. (1978) *Loss and Grief in Medicine*. London, Baillière Tindall.

Stewart J. (1979) *The Sexual Side of Handicap*. Cambridge, Woodhead Faulkner.

Tiffany R. (1980) *Oncology for Nurses and Health Care Professionals*, Vol. 1 & 2. London, George Allen & Unwin.

Wilson – Barnett J. (1979) *Stress in Hospital*. Edinburgh, Churchill Livingstone.

Index

Italicized page numbers indicate that the entry appears in a figure legend.

defects 34-7, 163
hypoplasia 25-6, 53
operations of 211-15
prolapse 30, 124-30
retroversion 122-4
'sedatives' for 167
spasms 26-7

Vacuum aspiration 168
Vagina
anatomy 72-4
carcinoma 75
cysts 75
cytology 97
defects 34-7
dilatation 177, 178, 179
discharge 25, 30-3
fistulae 75-7
operations of 216
packs for 8, 9, 128
pH 31, 48, 50, 72, 74, 159
preoperative care 7
prolapse 124, 125
senile vaginitis 74
smear 185
Vaginal urethoplasty 83
Vaginismus 179

Vasectomy 198
Venereal disease (VD) 79, 153
clinics 158-9
Venous thrombosis 5, 71
Ventrosuspension (Gilliam's) 124, 215
Vestibular bulbs 60
Vulva
anatomy 58-60
carcinoma 60, 61, 67-72
examination 18
herpes genitalis 65
hygiene 10, 33, 64, 65
operations of 216
pruritus vulvae 25, 60-2, 67
tumours 66-7

Warts, genital 66, 157
Wasserman reaction (WR) 133, 155
Weight loss 100, 110, 147, 149
Well Women Clinics 201-2
Wertheim's hysterectomy 101, 212
Wolffian ducts 34
'Womb stone' 113
Wound care 13
in radical vulvectomy 70-1

Zinc deficiency 164